Fit Kids for Life

A Parent's Guide to Optimal Nutrition & Training for Young Athletes

Jose Antonio, Ph.D.,
and Jeffrey R. Stout, Ph.D.

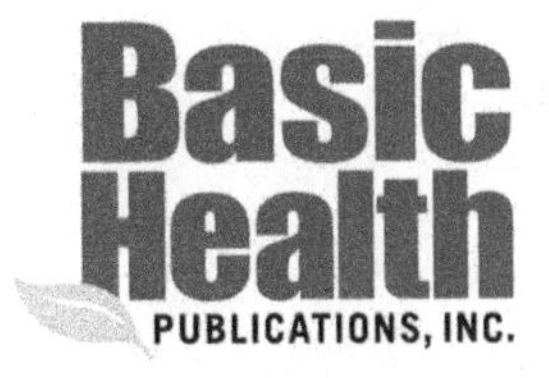

Basic Health Publications, Inc.

Library of Congress Cataloging-in-Publication Data

Antonio, Jose, PhD.
Fit kids for life : a parent's guide to optimal nutrition and training for young athletes / Jose Antonio and Jeffrey R. Stout.—1st ed.
p. cm.
Includes bibliographical references and index.

ISBN 978-1-59120-099-4 (Pbk.)
ISBN 978-1-68162-719-9 (Hardcover)

1. Teenagers—Nutrition. 2. Child athletes—Nutrition. 3. High school athletes—Nutrition. I. Stout, Jeffrey R. II. Title.

RJ235.A55 2004
613.7'11'083—dc22

2003023160

Editor: John Anderson
Typesetter/Book design: Gary A. Rosenberg
Cover design: Mike Stromberg
Photo credit: Mikey Gudikunst

Contents

To our wives,
Karla and Martha,
and our Fit Kids,
Brooke, Brandi,
Nicole, and Jeff

Foreword

As a family practice physician, I am aware of the expanding waistlines and all-around poor eating and exercise habits of most Americans. Sadly, not only is the average adult overweight and out of shape, but American children are fast becoming the most rotund and inactive kids in the world. Nevertheless, I applaud those parents who spend time with their children and teach them the value and utter necessity of exercise and good eating. *Fit Kids for Life* is an excellent, easy-to-read, and informative choice for parents who seek credible information that they want to pass along to their kids. Let's face it, there is nothing more important than the legacy you leave your child. If that includes healthy exercising and eating habits, then you deserve nothing but praise. I know that physicians, scientists, and parents will find *Fit Kids for Life* a great resource.

Eric Serrano, M.D.
Family Practice Physician
Columbus, Ohio

INTRODUCTION

Fit Kids Become Fit Adults

As adults, it becomes painfully clear to us that staying in shape requires work, discipline, and dedication. For some, exercise itself becomes a chore. But for others, exercise is as natural as brushing your teeth: you get up, you do it, and you don't think about it.

When we look back at childhood, we realize that exercise then was a lot like play. Recess was our favorite time at school: by running, playing tag or kickball, we "exercised" as kids. And if we were lucky enough, we carried these healthy habits into adulthood.

However, it's apparent that staying active, even as kids, has now become the exception rather than the rule. The statistics are depressing: up to 30 percent of children in the United States are obese. And that doesn't count kids who are sedentary, out-of-shape, and on their way to adult fatness.[1] In actuality, overweight kids become overweight adults. According to a report in *Health & Fitness Journal,* "approximately 40 percent of obese 7-year-old children and 70 percent of obese adolescents become obese adults." If this trend continues, by the year 2050, 75 percent of Americans will be overweight.[2]

The fact is that very few cases of childhood obesity are related to a genetic or hormonal defect. But the chances of overweight kids becoming overweight adults are much greater if their parents are also overweight. A recent general opinion poll found that two-

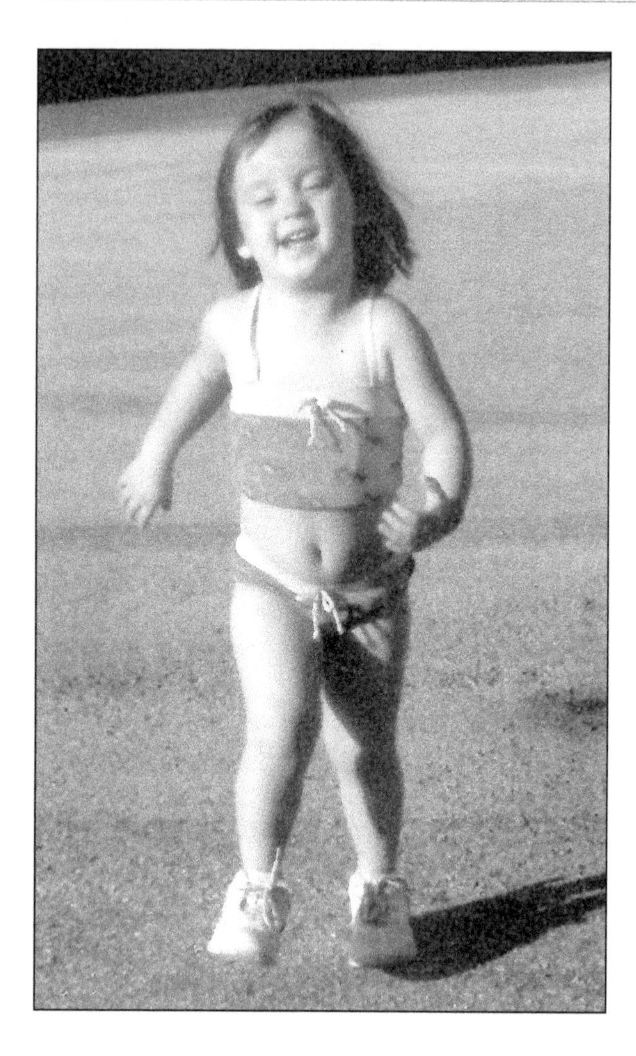

When we look back at childhood, we realize that exercise then was a lot like play.

thirds of people thought that parents or guardians bore the most responsibility for obesity in children (fast-food restaurants were second in the survey).[3] So, as parents, you can alter and control factors that might impact the fitness or fatness of your child.

If your child is participating in an exercise program, you've already won half the battle: your child will be much more likely to maintain such healthy habits into adulthood. The other half is establishing proper eating habits. This may be difficult, particularly because kids (as well as adults) associate food consumption with certain emotional states. Kids and adults eat to celebrate holidays and birthdays, when they're happy or depressed, when they're bored, and when they're watching television. If you can instill the importance of healthy and beneficial eating habits, you can permanently influence your child's behavior as an adult.

Don't let your children grow up to become obese. This book can show you how to help your kids become more active and eat right, so that your fit kids become fit adults.

EXERCISE AND SPORTS PARTICIPATION

Children usually play sports for the simple reason that they enjoy it. Parents, on the other hand, are often leery of the impact that exercise and sports may have on their child's development. However, research shows that kids who play sports tend to excel in school and have better social skills and higher self-esteem. Sports may also help prevent drug and alcohol abuse, and children who participate in sports are less likely to start smoking.

Furthermore, did you know that many of the risk factors for disease are already present in childhood? Lack of physical activity in children could lead to metabolic disorders, such as obesity, diabetes, and hypertension, that may not appear until adulthood. And childhood obesity, a precursor for heart disease, is on the rise. These risk factors can be diminished, or nearly eliminated, with regular physical exercise.

Weight training, as we will discuss in Part One, provides a myriad of physical benefits for kids, including stronger bones, enhanced strength, and improved athletic ability. Bones, ligaments, and muscles have been shown to respond favorably to the stresses placed upon them in weight training. Resistance training can also significantly improve strength in growing children, beyond what typically occurs during natural development.

THE IMPORTANCE OF NUTRITION

The more kids exercise and participate in sports, the more calories and nutrients they need. Athletics create more nutritional demands on the body, especially when a hectic and unhealthy eating schedule has become a habit. Parents and young athletes need to understand the importance of high-quality nutrition.

Whereas in the past there was a preoccupation with simply meeting a child's nutritional needs (the four food groups, vitamins, and so on), now there's a major shift toward the importance of how childhood nutrition will impact health much later in life. From eating habits themselves to preventing or encouraging disease, how your child eats today will have a striking impact on his or her health throughout adolescence and adulthood. After birth, with the exception of infancy, the human body grows the fastest during childhood and adolescence. This rapid growth makes proper nutrition an obligation and, without it, children may suffer harmful and irreversible effects on their permanent growth and development.

Physical activity also takes its toll. We already know kids need a lot of calories for proper growth, but sporting activities place tremendous demands on the respiratory, cardiovascular, muscular, and skeletal systems. This is especially important today when more kids, at younger ages than ever before, are participating in sports.

THE FIT KIDS FOR LIFE PLAN

This book provides exercise and nutrition guidelines for kids so that parents can help their children stay active and healthy.

In Part One, we discuss proper fitness training for young athletes. There are many common misconceptions regarding strength training for children. The fact is that kids *can* safely use resistance training to get fit for recreational activities and sports. This section covers:

- The benefits of exercise and sports
- Simple exercise rules
- Safe and effective weight-lifting techniques

Part Two offers healthy eating guidelines for active kids. You'll discover:

- How to provide a balanced and nutritious diet
- Sample meal plans and healthy snacking
- Pre- and postexercise eating guidelines
- How kids can stay hydrated while exercising
- How to help kids lose or gain weight safely

We hope that *Fit Kids for Life* will help keep your young athletes injury-free, active, and healthy right into adulthood.

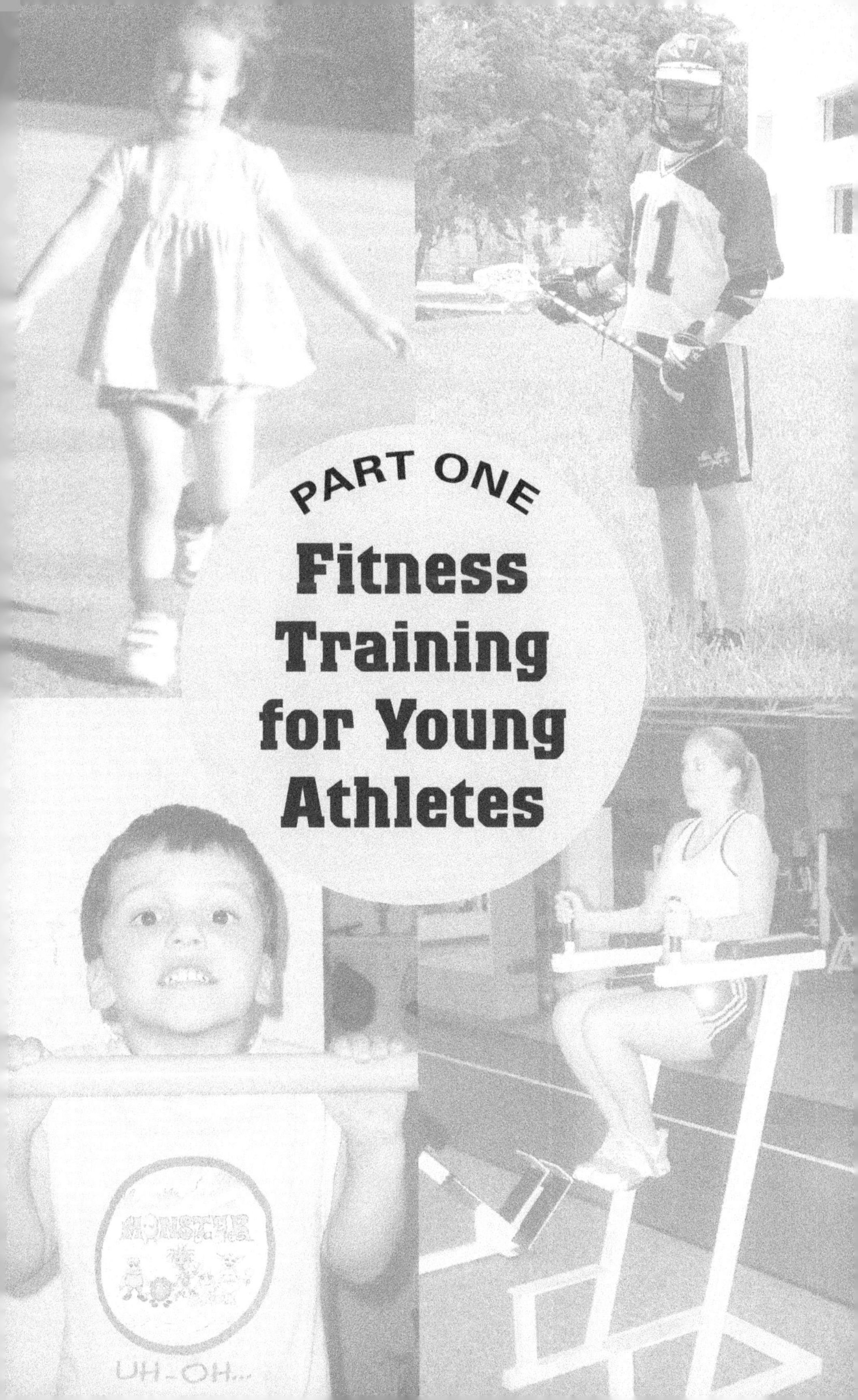

PART ONE

Fitness Training for Young Athletes

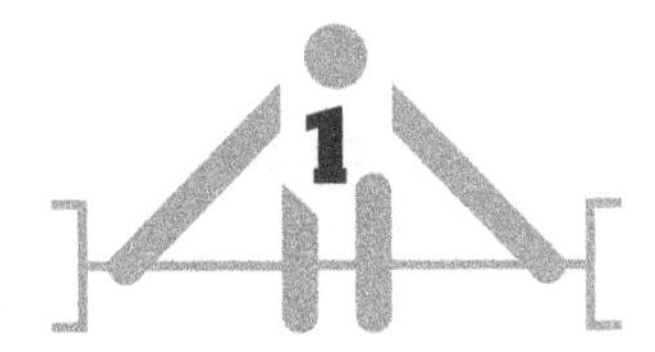

The Benefits of Exercise and Sports Participation for Kids

Any child in America today who decides to participate in sports usually does so for one simple reason: fun. Now, if only the decision was that elementary for parents, who are often unsure of the impact that exercise and sports may have on their child's physical development and academic achievement. Fortunately for parents, as research can attest, exercise and sports offer tremendous opportunities for social

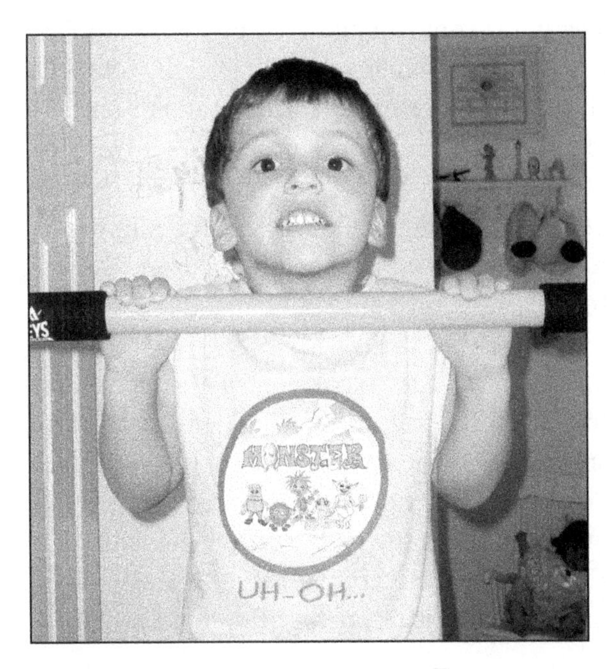

Participating in sports and exercise promotes a positive attitude toward activity that will likely continue into adulthood.

relationships, physical challenges, and honest competition. There is even evidence that sports can increase a child's self-esteem and academic performance, while decreasing the likelihood of disease and drug use.[1] Then again, to a child, all of these attributes equal just one desirable characteristic: fun.

Athletic participation and training for sports can provide a myriad of benefits that few other activities offer. But the burden of responsibility has increased for parents. We live in a lazy society and for many kids the word "sports" means playing video games. Today, leisure time for children is significantly less devoted to rigorous activities. The hardest part is just getting them to start exercising. On the bright side, research has also shown that participating in sports and exercise at a young age promotes a positive attitude toward activity that will likely continue into adulthood.

HEALTH PROMOTION AND DISEASE PREVENTION

It may be surprising to learn that many of the risk factors for heart disease are already present in childhood and early adolescence. Lack of physical activity in children could lead to metabolic disorders (obesity, diabetes, hypertension) that may not surface for decades. Childhood obesity, another precursor for heart disease, has increased by more than 50 percent since 1976. Fortunately, these risk factors can be diminished, or nearly eliminated, with regular physical exercise. For instance, in children who exercise, HDL cholesterol (the good kind) is elevated—a positive finding.[2]

Furthermore, with exercise the expansion of the body's fat cells is markedly reduced, decreasing the likelihood of obesity. The number of fat cells present in the body is determined in early adolescence; from that point on, we do not acquire or lose fat cells. So, the fat that is often gained later in life is due to those existing fat cells growing larger and larger. The crucial piece in this puzzle, and the key to avoiding fat gains, is to prevent the rapid prolifera-

Benefits of Exercise and Sports Participation

Health Promotion and Disease Prevention:

- Diminishes risk of childhood obesity
- Decreases likelihood of diabetes
- Decreases risk of hypertension
- Guards against osteoporosis
- Decreases risk of breast cancer

Social, Academic, and Psychological Benefits:

- Better grades in school
- Enhanced social skills
- Prevention of drug/alcohol abuse
- Decreased likelihood of smoking
- Increased self-esteem and confidence
- Healthier body image

Physical Benefits of Weight Training:

- Stronger bones
- Enhanced strength
- Improved athletic ability
- Increased power, speed, and agility
- Reduced chance of injury
- Enhanced recovery

tion of fat cells during childhood.[3] That way, there simply won't be as many cells with the potential to grow larger. Of course, the best way to keep your child's fat cell count as low as possible is to promote daily exercise and healthy eating habits. This will not only prevent obesity, but it will also stave off other diseases.

SOCIAL, ACADEMIC, AND PSYCHOLOGICAL BENEFITS

The benefits of exercise go beyond health. According to researchers at The Institute for the Study of Youth Sports at Michigan State University, kids who play sports actually do better in school and have enhanced social skills. Sports may also help prevent drug and alcohol abuse, and children who participate in sports are less likely to start smoking or, if they do smoke, are more likely to quit.[4]

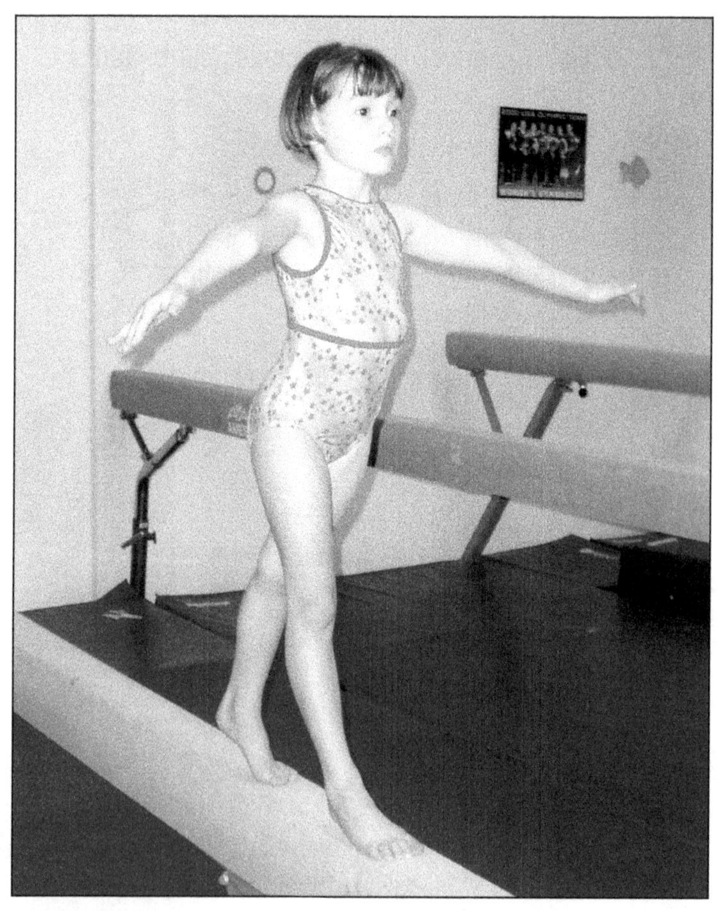

Participating in sports allows children to bond with teammates and to value the accomplishments of their bodies and minds.

Research on the benefits of sports and exercise for girls has been particularly promising. The President's Council on Physical Fitness and Sports has reported that athletically active girls develop increased self-esteem and confidence, are more likely to finish high school and college, and have a healthier body image.[5] The Women's Sports Foundation has also found that females participating in sports are less likely to become pregnant as teenagers and they suffer less depression.[6] Furthermore, there is evidence that athletic activity can decrease the likelihood of developing breast cancer and osteoporosis.[7] Fortunately for females, given the increased popularity of women's collegiate, professional, and Olympic sporting events, the opportunities to participate in sports as children are more promising than ever before.

Fortunately for females, given the increased popularity of women's collegiate, professional, and Olympic sporting events, the opportunities to participate in sports as children are more promising than ever before.

The social benefits of exercise and sports participation are almost too numerous to count. How can you possibly measure the value and satisfaction derived from working hard and mastering a skill? We've all done it, and the feeling is exhilarating, regardless of age. With sports and exercise, a child has the opportunity to experience this on almost a daily basis. On the same note, skill acquisition allows children to value the accomplishments of their bodies and minds, increasing confidence and making further challenges in life less daunting. These attributes simply can't be measured—neither can developing a sense of community through sports, bonding with new friends and teammates, and improving relationships with adults. Participating in sports also allows children to take on leadership roles, handle adversity, and improve their time management—qualities important for succeeding in adulthood.

PHYSICAL BENEFITS OF WEIGHT TRAINING

Some interesting new research is now uncovering the vast array of benefits provided by weight training, including stronger bones, enhanced strength, and improved athletic ability. However, when parents ask about the risks and benefits of weight training for children, they're always concerned about potential damage to bone growth. Sadly, this stems from a myth that weight lifting in children will lead to the premature closure of the end plates of long bones, thereby stunting their growth. In reality, any damage to these growth plates is usually a result of fractures that occur from repeated maximal lifts, lack of adult supervision, and improper lifting techniques. Overall, the risk of injury in children who train with weights is actually quite low, as long as appropriate training guidelines are followed.

For example, in a study that examined more than 1,500 sports injuries in children over a one-year period, only 0.7 percent of

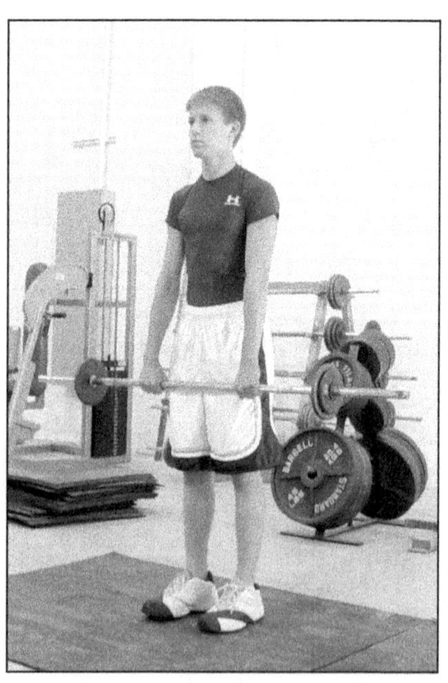

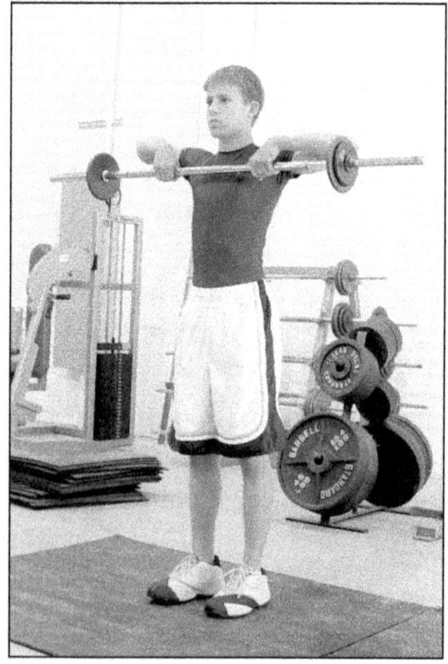

Studies have demonstrated a decreased injury rate in young athletes who have undergone weight training.

injuries were a result of weight training. Perhaps not surprisingly, football, wrestling, and gymnastics topped the list. Furthermore, researchers concluded that weight training is significantly safer than many other sports and activities.[8]

"The benefits of resistance training for kids resides in the fact that it promotes an active lifestyle and can help enhance the development of young bodies," argues William J. Kraemer, Ph.D., of the University of Connecticut. "With improvements in physiological function, physical capabilities, prevention of sports injuries, and improved sports performance, resistance training is a safe and effective exercise modality. It is also important that children prepare their bodies for the rigors of sport and recreational activity. Finally, fighting the negative effects of aging starts when you are young and resistance training plays a vital role."

The benefits of resistance training for kids resides in the fact that it promotes an active lifestyle and can help enhance the development of young bodies. . . . resistance training is a safe and effective exercise modality.

—WILLIAM J. KRAEMER, PH.D., UNIVERSITY OF CONNECTICUT

Interestingly, proper weight training and exercise can actually improve bone strength. Bones, ligaments, and muscles are dynamic connective tissues that respond favorably to the stresses placed upon them.[9] Certainly you've heard the phrase "use it or lose it." That essentially describes bone: the more you "pound" it, the stronger it becomes. For example, researchers in the Netherlands have reported that high-impact strength training and explosive exercise, such as skipping, running, and jumping, are more effective for bone development than activities like walking, bicycling, and swimming. They concluded that bone responds best to exercise characterized by unexpected high loads of relatively short duration. This is, in fact, exactly what takes place in

The Benefits and Pitfalls of Sports Specialization

One of the more difficult decisions a parent has to make regarding a child's athletic participation involves sports specialization—the practice of focusing increased time, instruction, and training on one specific sport. From Olympic hopefuls to golfer Tiger Woods, specialization has made superstar athletes out of high-school students. Many even begin their chosen sport as toddlers. And while a select few go on to fame and fortune, many more suffer from injuries or burnout. It's simply impossible to forecast whether a child's talents are prolific enough to thrive at the professional level one day. Nevertheless, specialization via "elite" coaching and clubs is probably here to stay.

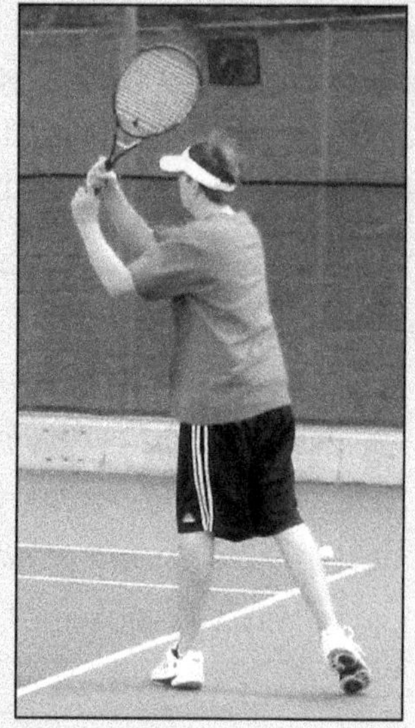

But there's question as to whether specialization even works. And if it does, is it logical to specialize when only a handful of athletes will ever achieve professional success? Researchers have stated

sports such as baseball, football, and basketball. Researchers went so far as to espouse weight-bearing activity and high-impact strength training for both boys and girls, citing the fact that the earlier a child starts with physical activity, the more bone that's accumulated.[10]

There is no shortage of data to support the conclusion that

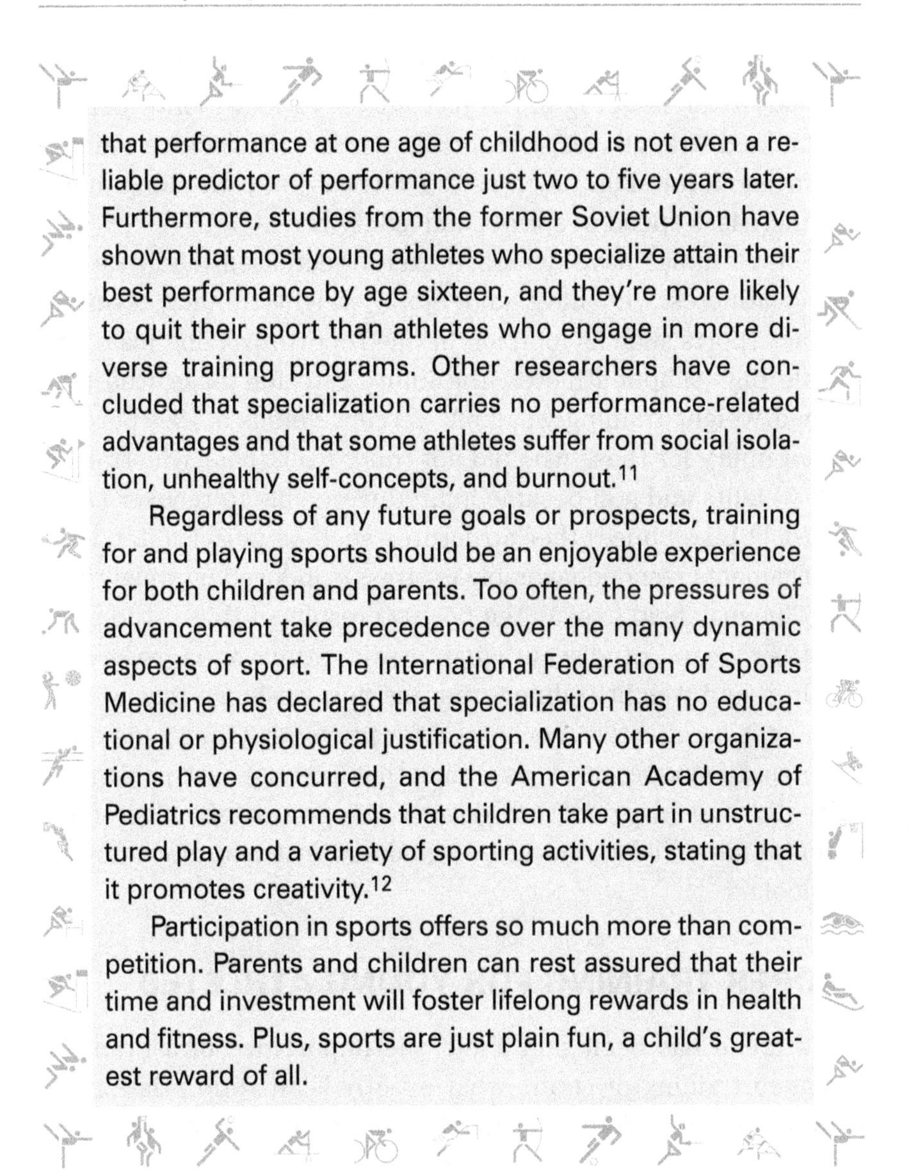

that performance at one age of childhood is not even a reliable predictor of performance just two to five years later. Furthermore, studies from the former Soviet Union have shown that most young athletes who specialize attain their best performance by age sixteen, and they're more likely to quit their sport than athletes who engage in more diverse training programs. Other researchers have concluded that specialization carries no performance-related advantages and that some athletes suffer from social isolation, unhealthy self-concepts, and burnout.[11]

Regardless of any future goals or prospects, training for and playing sports should be an enjoyable experience for both children and parents. Too often, the pressures of advancement take precedence over the many dynamic aspects of sport. The International Federation of Sports Medicine has declared that specialization has no educational or physiological justification. Many other organizations have concurred, and the American Academy of Pediatrics recommends that children take part in unstructured play and a variety of sporting activities, stating that it promotes creativity.[12]

Participation in sports offers so much more than competition. Parents and children can rest assured that their time and investment will foster lifelong rewards in health and fitness. Plus, sports are just plain fun, a child's greatest reward of all.

resistance training can significantly improve strength in children, well beyond what typically occurs during natural development. This is apparent even in children as young as five years old! In a recent study, five to twelve year olds underwent an eight-week strength-training program. The results demonstrated increases in strength of 30 to 40 percent.[13] Furthermore, strength gains of roughly 30 to 50 percent can be expected (in boys and girls) with a quality exercise program in just a two- to four-month period. That added strength isn't just for show, either. Resistance training improves motor skills, such as the vertical jump and long jump, and increases speed in sprints and agility runs.[14]

Some studies have demonstrated a decreased injury rate in young athletes who have undergone weight training, even in contact sports such as football. In one report involving male and female high-school athletes, the injury rate for those who performed weight training was 26.2 percent versus a 72.4 percent rate of injury for those who did not train. Also, those who trained with weights and still became injured were able to recover twice as fast.[15] Like bone, other structures such as muscles, tendons, and ligaments respond favorably to stresses induced by weight lifting. This may help explain the positive results of these studies.

After years of discouraging media propaganda regarding children and weight training, there is now evidence that weight training is an effective mechanism for preventing injury in young athletes. Of course, this is assuming that exercises are performed correctly and programs are designed appropriately. Therefore, parental supervision and use of qualified instructors cannot be overlooked.

PROPER TRAINING FOR YOUNG ATHLETES

Since much has been said about the importance of a properly designed training program, what exactly is an appropriate regimen for young athletes? Although that's a complicated question, some basic tenets can be outlined.

First of all, it should be stated that the most common injuries among children who weight train are joint strains and muscle strains of the low back. While this is likely due to poor technique, it may also stem from a lack of "core" training. Core training should be a top priority in young athletes who wish to lift weights. It involves general strengthening of the muscles surrounding the abdomen and low back. This is the "hub" or base of operations for

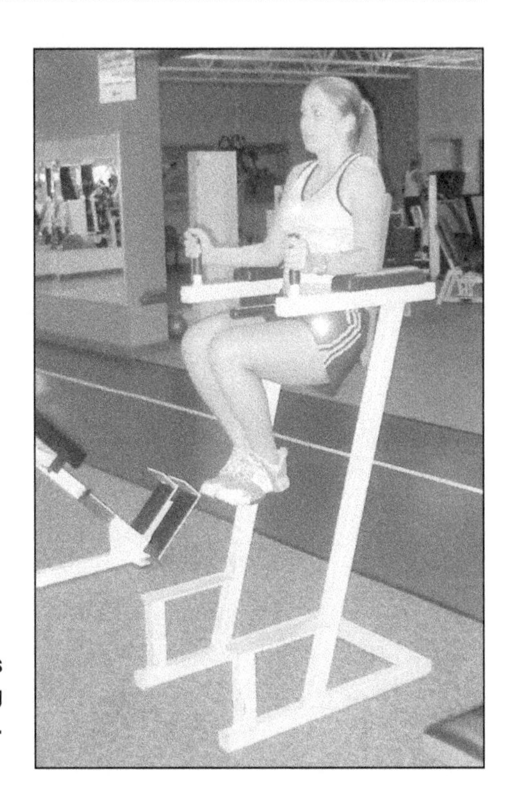

Abdominal training is important for building core strength.

the extremities; without a strong core, muscle imbalances and injury are more likely. Also, core development is extremely important for sports because power traveling from the legs to the upper body, or vice versa, must be transferred by the core muscles. By the way, this transfer occurs when playing nearly *every* sport, so core training is mandatory.

When a child is mentally and physically ready to engage in weight training, exercises need to focus on proper technique—keeping the weight moderate and using a high number of repetitions (10–20). The entire body should be trained to promote balance, maximal loads should be avoided, and stretching and calisthenics must be incorporated.

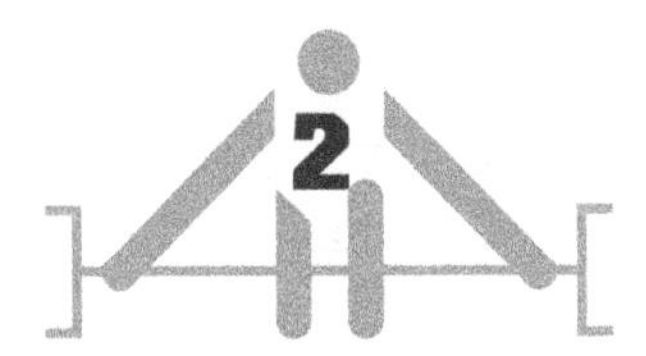

Simple Rules of Exercise for Kids

Research shows that it is safe for children to lift weights and exercise. It will not, as rumored, stunt their growth, break their bones, fill them with rage, or abruptly and profoundly drop their IQ. A child who lifts weights can still take part in intellectual pursuits, finish his or her homework, or become a computer whiz. And weight training and working out may actually help improve performance in these areas. No, not in a "bigger biceps will make them a stronger artist" sort of way—rather, pumping iron and becoming fit can do wonders for a child's self-esteem and confidence, and it will add to their energy reserves and motivation, not detract from them. Plus, stronger muscles can make a child a better athlete.

So, let's get something straight right from the get-go: weight lifting, when done correctly, is not dangerous. In fact, it's quite healthy and has been shown to reduce the prevalence of injury, both in the weight room and out on the field of play.[1] Do not surrender yourself to the myth that lifting weights is dangerous for your children, regardless of what many conventional doctors may claim. Studies have repeatedly shown that poor technique and lifting habits lead to injury, whether you're nine or thirty-nine.[2] Proper exercise training can set your kid off on the right foot for a lifetime of growth (inner *and* outer) and achievement.

To begin, let's keep the rules of exercise for kids simple and straightforward—no advanced training techniques, secret potions, or web of convoluted directions, which they don't need. A thirty-year-old exercise fanatic who has performed the same exercises for most of his life may need new direction and creativity, but your child does not. Good, sound advice on how to work out safely and effectively is all children require to get going. They'll get stronger (and maybe shed some baby fat) by adhering to the following rules.

RULE 1: FOCUS ON THE CORE AND THEN EXPAND OUTWARD

A growing tree is nothing without the trunk, and its branches can't be considered powerful without a strong attachment to the base. Likewise, the trunk of a child is the center of all operations, and any weakness here will make big arms and legs useless. The

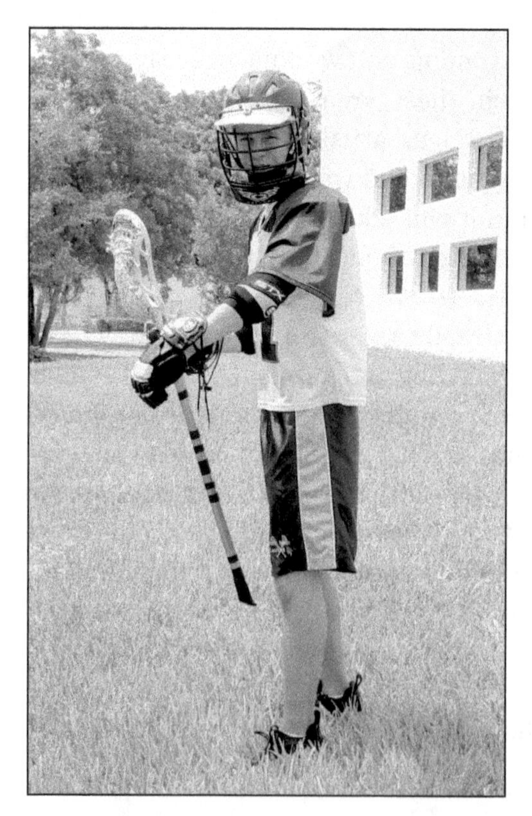

Beyond allowing the extremities to develop their true power, core strength is crucial in nearly every sport.

abdominal and low back area, also known as "the core," is extremely important in providing the base of support that allows the extremities (arms and legs) to be used efficiently. Of course, this is true of any age group. We've seen countless weight lifters who can't even perform a squat with their own body weight because they lack the coordination and core strength that together allow maximum potential from their legs. Don't let this happen to your child.

Beyond allowing the extremities to develop their true power, core strength is crucial in nearly every sport. In most cases, the arms and legs of those playing baseball, basketball, tennis, golf, soccer, football, hockey, lacrosse, and so on, are simply the last link in the fitness chain. For example, take swinging a baseball bat, tennis racket, or hockey stick. In all these activities the final motion is in the arms, but the power for the movement arises from the legs and is transferred through the body—passing through the core—upward to the arms. If the core is strong, it's the checkered flag; if not, it's a traffic jam and the power can't get through.

The core is the first area of the body that needs to be trained, but how do you do it? Well, some of the best techniques involve the use of a medicine ball. This weighted ball is terrific for providing the momentum that serves as resistance for the abdominal muscles. Start out light (2–3 pounds for beginners ages eight to ten; 3–5 pounds for those ten to twelve years old; 5–8 pounds for young adolescents) and work your way up. For example, have your child stand ready with knees and hips bent and hands ready to catch (the athletic pose), and toss the ball to the sides of his or her body. Your child should only rotate the trunk while catching the ball, thereby making the abdominal muscles do the work. Have your child throw it back in the same manner. This is great for kids to do with one another. Then they can mix in shuffling side to side while catching the ball, sitting back to back and performing rotating hand-offs, and catching a ball two-handed above their heads. Of course, there's a litany of exercises, so seek out a qualified trainer to teach them more.

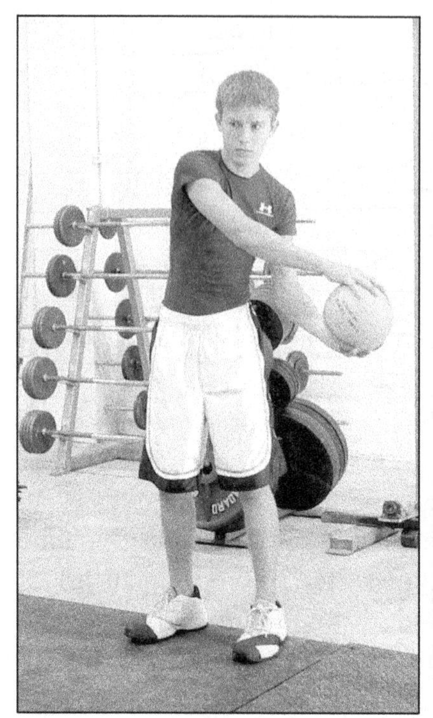

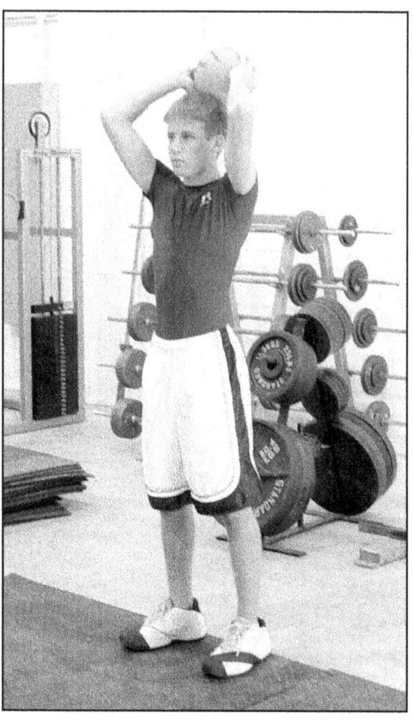

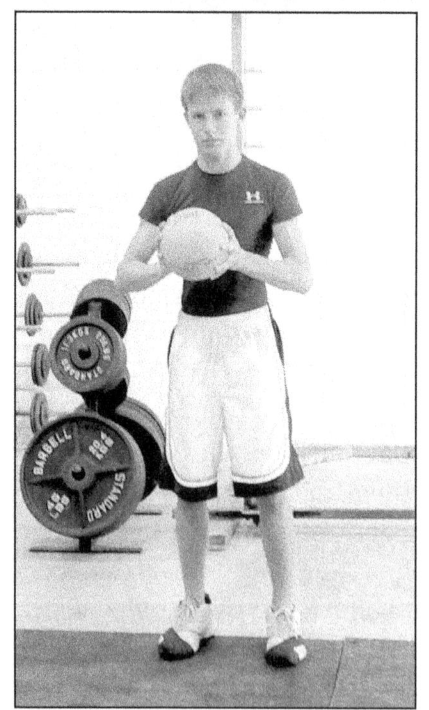

Medicine ball workout.

Performing side-to-side, forward, and overhead movements and throws with a medicine ball is important for improving shoulder, chest, and core strength.

There are also traditional floor abdominal exercises. Sit-ups and crunches are effective, but they are highly overrated. It's better to have your child lie down on his or her back, keeping the back flat as a pancake on the floor with the stomach tucked in, and then perform any of the numerous exercises that lead to a strong core. From this position, the child can raise his or her legs straight up in the air and then lower them slowly to the ground while keeping the back flat and abdominal muscles tight. They can also perform scissor exercises (crossing and uncrossing the legs in the air) while maintaining core position. Again, there are many variations, so consult a good trainer or book of exercises, such as *Strength and Power for Young Athletes* by A. Faigenbaum and W. Westcott (see Resources).

This type of training should be performed three to four times per week for about twenty minutes. Each set of medicine ball or floor exercises should initially last between thirty and forty-five seconds, but can be increased to three to five minutes at a time to improve endurance.

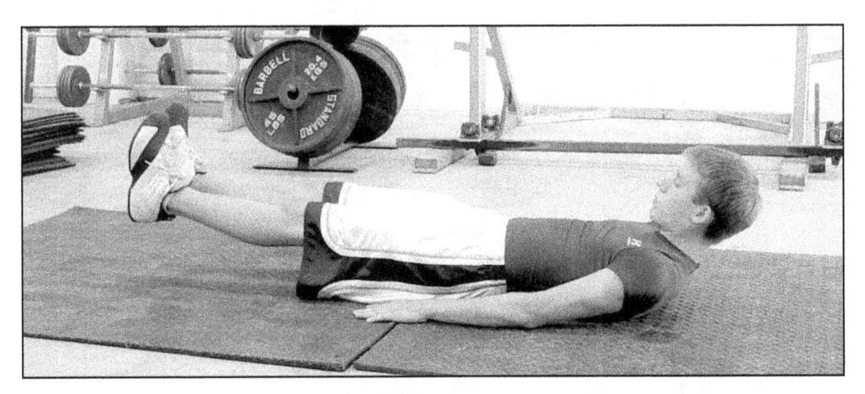

Leg lift exercise.

RULE 2: DON'T NEGLECT AGILITY AND BALANCE

Too many kids want to jump feet first into the deep end of the exercising pool and skip right to lifting heavy weights. Well, if patience is a virtue, parents will need to exercise a bit of their own to keep their kids' egos from invading their workout regi-

Family Involvement Is Important

We've witnessed many out-of-shape parents dropping off their kids at soccer, gymnastics, or baseball practice. Clearly, it would be much better if the parents also exercised and were in shape—the *best* role model for a child is a fit parent. But the second-best solution is for the not-so-fit parent to provide emotional support for the child who participates in sports.

For instance, one study showed that with boys and girls in the fifth and sixth grades variables such as the mother's attitude, and support from friends and family influenced exercise behavior.[3] This clearly indicates the need for emotional support for childhood activity and that the lack of support might promote a negative or apathetic attitude toward exercise.

Lead by example: if you're an active parent, there are ways to be more participatory (and less of a spectator) in

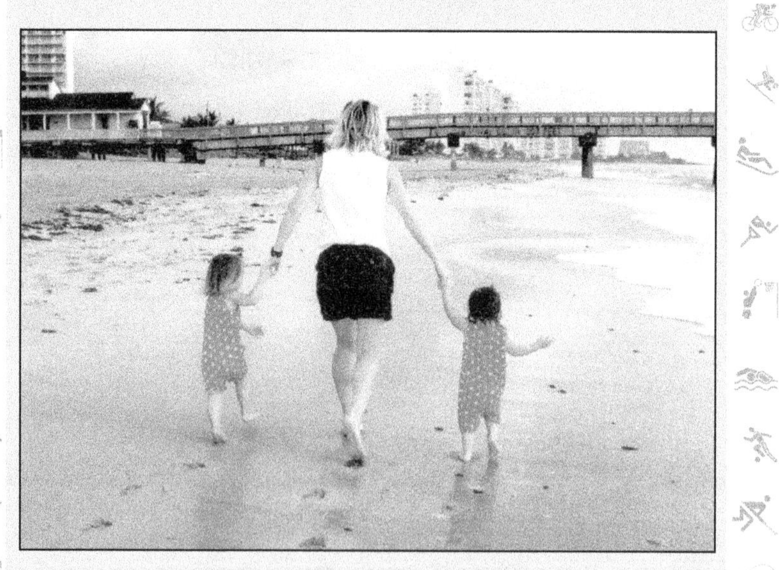

Get involved with your kids' fitness.

your child's activities. For instance, if your child wants to lift weights, help him or her get sound advice from a certified personal trainer, and then work out with your child. You may want to consider taking family vacations that involve strenuous activities, such as white-water rafting or hiking. Or if your child wants to practice soccer kicks, go out on the field and participate. The same applies to baseball, football, and most other sports.

Research has demonstrated that kids are much more likely to exercise if their parents exercise.[4] For example, when parents participate in their children's activities rather than just commanding them to be active, the kids tended to be more active.[5] However, parental inactivity is strongly related to sedentary behavior in kids.[6] Family involvement and socialization are vital to kids' physical exercise patterns.

Bottom line: It's better to be a player than an onlooker.

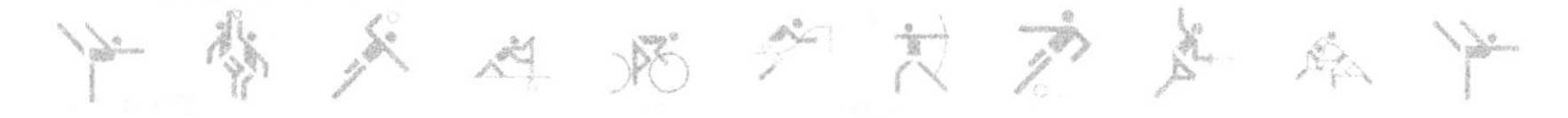

mens. With core strength developed first, kids can then graduate to some quicker, more challenging movements that improve agility, speed, power, and balance. All of these attributes are crucial in playing sports: the champions are rarely the strongest, and how much you can bench-press is of little consequence on the playing field. Proper agility and balance training is a must.

Side-to-side shuffling, single-leg hops, diagonal jumps, standing on one leg while playing catch, lunge jumps, sprints, walking on hands while a partner holds the legs, jumping rope, and running with rapid changes of direction are all fantastic methods for improving agility and balance. You can even mix in some medicine ball work. For example, have a child perform explosive jumps onto an 18-inch box or bench while catching a lightweight medicine ball to his or her side upon landing. You're only limited by your imagination and there are plenty of resources for these types of exercises.

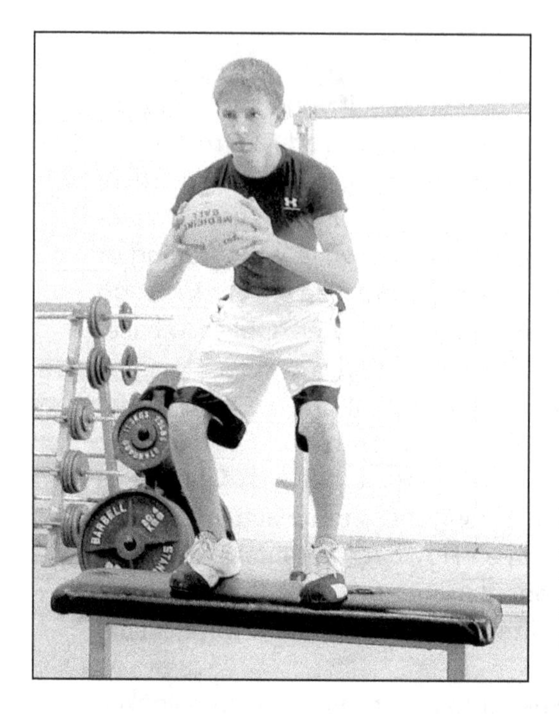

Explosive jumps onto a bench while catching a lightweight medicine ball improves agility and balance.

These exercises should be performed three to four times a week. Keep the rules the same as with the core training: twenty to thirty minutes, starting out with sets of thirty to forty-five seconds, and gradually increasing the minutes.

RULE 3: NOW IT'S TIME TO HIT THE WEIGHTS

Until a child has performed at least six weeks of core and agility/ balance training, incorporating traditional weight- (or resistance-) training exercises is not necessary. In reality, this type of exercise requires less coordination and proficiency than the agility and balance drills, and it has less specificity to bona fide sports. Nevertheless, it's extremely important and can make monumental improvements in the sporting lives of children. Furthermore, weight lifting will have the most profound and lasting effects on their growing bodies. Put simply, the weight room is where muscles are born.

Exercises should focus primarily on those movements that

encompass a number of muscles at once: squats, lunges, bench press, overhead press, pull-ups, rows, and all their variations. Additional exercises like biceps curls and hamstring curls, triceps extensions, and other isolation movements should be placed at the end of the training session and thus carry less significance. A child's body should grow as a whole, not look like its parts have been stuck together like pieces from a junkyard; therefore, it should be trained holistically. (See Chapter 3 for more detailed information on specific workouts.)

In weight training, proper technique is crucial. Performing each exercise through the correct range of motion will ensure that the child's muscles will gain strength and flexibility. A child should never be left to train alone in the weight room; adult supervision is mandatory, and instruction from a qualified trainer will be necessary. Every high school should have a trainer on staff, and younger children can be taught these exercises through private or group lessons run by coaches. Remember, with proper technique, children can reduce the likelihood of injury in the sporting arena.

Three to five sets of different exercises (5–7 lifts) per session is more than enough. Just keep the number of repetitions high (10 to 15 reps) and focus on strict form, not maxing out or exercising until their faces turn blue. Try three to four days per week of sessions lasting forty-five to sixty minutes. Or, more sensibly, a consolidated sixty-to-seventy-five-minute jam session that includes stretching followed by a combination of agility/balance, core, and weight-training drills.

RULE 4: TRAIN THE TICKER FOR INCREASED CARDIOVASCULAR ENDURANCE

There's no more pathetic sight than a bulked-up bodybuilder, who looks to be in fantastic shape but is doubled over in a fit of labored breathing after running half a block to catch the bus. The point is that looks mean nothing and give no indication of the true fitness of an individual. High-repetition weight training and agility

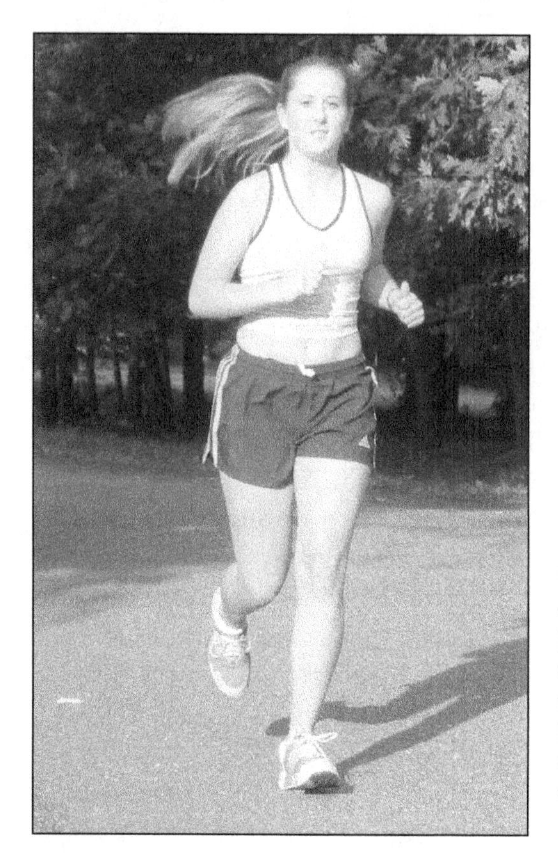

Regular endurance or cardiovascular training is important for strengthening the heart muscle, maintaining healthy bones, and enhancing overall well-being.

drills will improve the strength of the heart and cardiovascular endurance, but not as well as good old-fashioned running.

Thirty minutes of vigorous endurance exercise—running, cycling, stair-climbing, or other aerobic activity—performed three or more days per week will do wonders for the fitness and health of your child and will help reduce body fat as well. A person's adult body is formed and developed during childhood and adolescence, so keeping the fat at bay during these years will have lasting effects on your child's body composition.

RULE 5: PLAY!

Remember playing dodge ball, freeze tag, and kickball? Back in childhood, exercise was play. And it's still true that exercise just isn't fun if there's not some element of play involved. Kids are more likely to stick with an exercise program or sporting activity if they're having fun doing it.

So, add exercise to your play and play to your exercise. Encourage your child to participate in sports; for example, playing soccer can improve your child's endurance and agility, and basketball can improve his or her coordination and power. And make exercise fun with friendly competition, challenges, and variety. You already know that kids generally have short attention spans, so play according to their interests and also include yourself—you are not excused from exercise.

Finally, remember to visit a physician before your child starts engaging in any exercise regimen, and find a qualified instructor to show your child proper techniques. Keep the level of variety high and keep it fun. Children today face enough pressure with academics, so they don't need recreation to become another brick in the road to burnout. Rather, keep the fire of achievement and growth burning bright!

A SAMPLE WORKOUT ROUTINE

Here is a sample general workout routine for your child (and you) to begin with. The core and strength-training program should be done twice per week, along with endurance training three times per week. Enjoy, and good luck.

Stretching

Warm up for five to seven minutes with light jogging or biking. Then stretch major muscle groups of the chest, arms, hips, legs, and ankles.

Core Training + Agility/Balance

Perform three 45-second sets for each of the following exercises:

- Side-to-side shuffling with medicine ball catch/throw

- Single-leg diagonal hops with medicine ball catch/throw
- Box jumps with lightweight medicine ball catch
- Walking on hands with body balanced on a Swiss ball (also known as a stability ball; a large ball used to activate core muscles while performing various exercises)
- Leg raises and scissor kicks with stable abdomen and back lying flat on the floor

Weight Training

Perform three 10-to-15-rep sets for each of these exercises:

- Squats
- Lunges
- Bench press
- Pull-ups
- Flexed arm hang (hold position for 10–15 seconds)
- Leg extension
- Leg curls
- Upright row
- Shoulder press

For a complete description of how to do these exercises properly, see Chapter 3 and consult a personal trainer who is certified by the National Strength and Conditioning Association (see the website www.nsca-lift.org to locate a trainer near you).

Endurance

Running, biking, or other endurance activity or game; perform for twenty to thirty minutes.

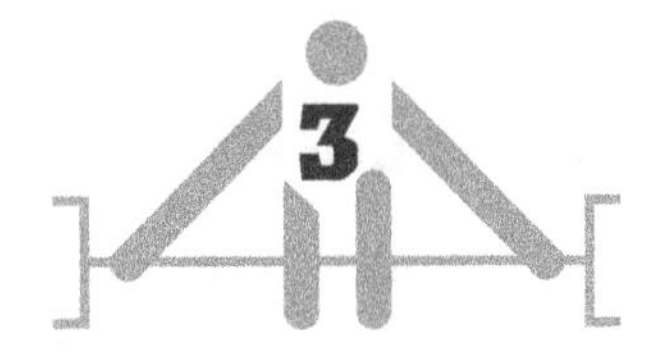

Strength Training and Conditioning for Kids

Contributed by Joel Raether, M.A.Ed., and Michael S. Sanders, M.A.Ed., CSCS

Running and weight training—in a nutshell, these are the two main components of an effective exercise program. We know running is generally considered good for you, but what about weight lifting?

- Does weight training stunt growth? This is actually a myth.
- Will lifting weights injure a child? Not if it is done safely with proper supervision and training.
- At what age can my child start lifting weights? The simple answer is—at any age that he or she wants, as long as adult supervision is present. Take, for instance, the age at which girls start gymnastics: often as young as two years old! Gymnastics is similar to weight training, except that in gymnastics you lift your body weight rather than a barbell, dumbbell, or other implement. But always remember, safety should be the main concern when considering weight lifting for your child.

This chapter will examine some of the common misconceptions regarding strength training for children, as well as look at developmental considerations, injury concerns, and program design. It will discuss coaching children, clarify gender-specific concerns surrounding strength training for children, and provide sample training programs.

THE TRUTH ABOUT WEIGHT TRAINING

For years, the issue of strength training for children has been clouded by uncertainties and gray area, leaving many parents with little guidance on how to improve performance and prevent injury. We've all heard the misconception that strength training is harmful for kids, that it causes long-term damage and is unsafe. In reality, these claims are unsupported. What comes as a surprise to most parents is that activities like running and jumping—things your child probably performs on a daily basis—likely stress the body to a greater extent than weight training, and tend to result in more frequent injuries. Of course, no one is demanding that children avoid these activities, but the point supports the view that strength training, when performed correctly, will not stunt your child's growth or increase risk of injury.

Today, it is known that strength training for children can be done safely, and moreover, strength training can enhance local muscular strength, improve performance, and diminish the possibility of injury during recreational activities. Most cases of injury to children from strength training occur from overhead lifts, attempting too much weight, or using poor technique. Additionally, poor supervision has been noted in these cases. This, of course, emphasizes the importance of paying attention to specific details and precautions before implementing a strength-training program for your child.

IS YOUR CHILD READY FOR STRENGTH TRAINING?

A professional, whether a physical educator or strength and conditioning coach, should consider a number of factors before training your child. For instance, he or she should determine your child's chronological and developmental age, level of physical maturity, prior strength-training experience, and degree of motor/muscular skill. These considerations will allow your child to achieve better skill acquisition and strength progression while creating a safe learning environment. The emphasis for strength training with children should not be directed toward lifting heavy loads but toward learning proper technique, making individual gains, and having fun in a healthy and playful atmosphere.

When assessing the chronological age and maturation of children, some general guidelines can be used. Both boys and girls show fairly linear increases in muscular strength until about the age of twelve or thirteen. From this point on, a boy's muscular strength increases drastically with the onset of puberty and the presence of anabolic hormones such as testosterone. Peak muscle mass in boys occurs between the ages of eighteen and twenty-five, whereas girls peak between the ages of sixteen and twenty. Most of the increases in muscular strength in preadolescents can be attributed to neural factors such as coordination and activation of more muscle fibers.

This means that training responses of boys and girls before the age of twelve or thirteen are similar due to physical similarities in strength and maturation. Following the onset of puberty, boys show much greater gains in muscular strength than girls, which would warrant different training expectations based on gender. While program considerations for boys and girls should remain the same after the onset of puberty, boys should begin to make larger strength gains because of the presence of anabolic hormones. Girls will continue to make gains, but not at the same rate as boys.

For both boys and girls, as the level of physical maturity advances, levels of motor control (coordination and skill development) and skill acquisition will also advance. There are three consecutive levels of learning skills: the novice or cognitive phase, followed by the intermediate or associative phase, and, lastly, the autonomous phase.[1] Each advance in motor skill will demonstrate higher levels of control and precision of movement, so much so that physical educators, coaches, and parents will readily observe noticeable changes. These changes may include a higher proficiency of movement, completion of higher numbers of repetitions with a given weight, and ease of transition to more advanced exercises and drills.

Children will go through all three of these phases, but the duration of each phase varies from child to child. For example, some children may only take a few weeks to advance from the novice phase to the intermediate phase, while others of the same age may take months to acquire intermediate skills. As your child's motor skills advance, so should the level of training. This match of training status with maturation will ensure that your child makes continual training gains.

BONE AND MUSCLE DEVELOPMENT

Along with motor development comes bone maturation and an increase in muscle size, a much anticipated badge of honor for the arduous work performed by your child. Of course, the extent of muscular growth in children is smaller than in adults because of the lower level of anabolic hormones present in children. But certainly the formation of new bone is a favorable offshoot and is perhaps more important, and acquired to a greater extent, than muscle growth. "Bone modeling," or the development of new bone material, is initiated by outside forces and impacts, such as weight training. When strength training is used with children, formation of new and stronger bone is a likely result. This development of new bone allows your child to withstand higher degrees of impact in recreational activities and also enables him or her to support larger loads during training.

So much for the belief that weight training damages bones! The issue of epiphyseal plate (EP) damage has brought much attention to the topic of children and strength training and, unfortunately, only in recent years has the controversy dissolved. Epiphyseal plates, or growth plates, are located at the ends of long bones, and they account for a bone's lengthening until the onset of puberty, at which point they ossify (harden and prevent further growth). It used to be thought that weight training would cause these endplates to ossify prematurely, thus stunting a child's growth. We now know this to be false but, nevertheless, before puberty these plates are vulnerable to fractures due to the portion of the bone that has yet to ossify. This can occur with weight training, though it is more likely in contact sports. Furthermore, reports of fractures to the plates have usually involved overhead lifts, as stated earlier.

It is important to note that the peak time for epiphyseal plate fracture occurs near the peak height growth stage, which in boys occurs between the ages of twelve and fourteen. Generally, girls will reach bone maturity two to three years before boys. Thus, one could argue that preadolescent children are at less risk of EP fractures compared with adolescent boys and girls. Moreover, any strength training your child undergoes during this vulnerable period should be closely monitored and possibly altered to ensure safety.

There have also been concerns about damage to growth cartilage from weight training. Growth cartilage can be found at the joint surfaces, tendon insertions, and the epiphyseal plates. These growth sites ensure stable connections from bone to tendon as well as act as shock absorbers between bone surfaces. Any damage to these sites may cause rough articulations between joints and possible separations of bone-to-tendon connections. However, damage to growth cartilage, bone fractures, and muscular strains are actually uncommon with strength-training activities.[2]

DEVELOPING A TRAINING PROGRAM

Before developing a resistance-training program for a child, we should take a few things into consideration. First, it is important to remember that the child is just that—a child. Children are not concerned with winning at all costs; rather, they want to have fun and experience something new and exciting. If a healthy and fun atmosphere is not created, children will tend to lose interest and quit training. Second, the physical educator or strength and conditioning coach should speak with the child to find out how he or she feels about the program. Is he or she having fun? Does it scare the child? Is it too hard? Also, is the child in a safe environment? Is the child being supervised correctly? The most important program considerations are the need for proper technique and a high level of supervision. The higher the coach-to-participant ratio, the greater the chances of learning correct training technique and the lower the chances of injury during training. The emphasis of the program should not be on how much weight is lifted, but on the development of lifting proficiency with all lifts and having fun with training.

Finally, your child's program should start off using very basic techniques with a low volume of weight and low intensity. As he or she grows older, the program should progressively become more difficult using increasingly complicated exercises, more volume, and higher intensities. This is probably the most difficult task for the physical educator or coach—to identify the best time to progress to the next level with the child safely and efficiently. We suggest starting the child in a strength-training program with basic multi-joint lifts, core strength training, flexibility training, and balance and agility drills (any training professional will have knowledge of these exercises). The chronological age of the child is less important than his or her physiological age (or training age). Motor skills, balance, posture, flexibility, and strength levels should be considered when deciding what a child needs and when he or she should progress further into a strength-training program. Remember that not all children are created equal in terms of movement skills. Regardless of age, all of these factors should be taken into account.

Another consideration that may not be as frequently discussed is the psychological status of the child to be trained. Is the child at a level at which he or she can listen effectively and apply coaching strategies? Does the child understand the importance of safety and the necessity of technique in training? If the physical educator, strength coach, or parent does not feel the child has these qualities, it might be best to wait until these qualities develop before entering the child into a training regimen. It is critical that parents are involved in their child's training program so that they can monitor the child's progress and ensure that he or she is receiving proper instruction in technique and safety.

When starting a strength-training program, all children should begin at a basic level, whatever their age. For example, if your child starts resistance training at age five, he or she should start with basic lifts using the guidelines above. However, if he or she doesn't start a weight-training program until the age of ten, still start at the same level as the five-year-old and take him or her through the same progressive steps.

One last consideration is sport-specific training. Resistance training can definitely increase your child's physical ability and protect him or her from injury in whatever sport he or she wants to play. It should be remembered, however, that a trainer is only trying to get a child interested in resistance training and improve the child physically. With that in mind, sport-specific training should be put on the back burner at the onset of training. The physical educator or strength coach might develop programs that are more sport-specific as the child grows older and shows proficiency and progress in his or her training.

Be sure that your child consults a physician for a general checkup before getting involved in training. And teach your child basic knowledge of injury prevention: for instance, muscle strain is the most common form of acute injury, and this type of injury is often sustained from improper or inadequate warm-up. A dynamic warm-up is therefore very beneficial, and may include slow jogging, skipping, light jumping, or even a game of light intensity. Next, a flexibility program should be employed, which will further increase intramuscular temperature and blood flow to working muscles and joints. If a proper warm-up is performed prior to each training session, the occurrence of muscle strain may be greatly diminished.

GUIDELINES AND SAMPLE TRAINING PROGRAMS FOR CHILDREN

The following are sample strength-training programs for children of different ages. These programs should not last longer than twenty to sixty minutes per session. Bear in mind that the following programs are not the only ways to train a child—there really is no best program. Use the training tips along with the preceding considerations to develop the best possible program for your child. Furthermore, each child will progress at a different rate due to differences in physical, neutral, and emotional maturity.

Training Age: Five Years and Under

Training Tips

- Communicate with the child to find out the level of interest in resistance training.
- Introduce simple movements using little or no weight. Broomsticks and dowel rods work well in place of heavy bars. Introduce the child to training-session basics, such as sets, repetitions, and goals.
- Show the child how to warm up and perform the exercises with proper technique. Technique is the prime focus at this point.

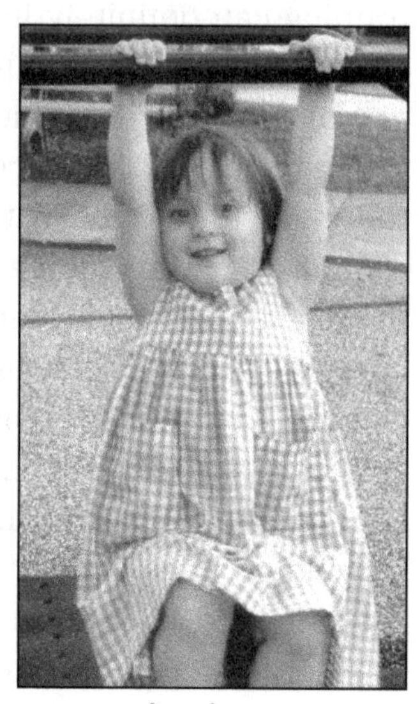

Arm hang.

- Be sure the child is able to handle the workload.
- Check flexibility, motor skills, strength, balance, and posture to be sure the child is in a safe range.
- Always emphasize technique and safety!

Sample Basic Training Session

Body-weight squats—Perform squats using just body weight with hands on hips to maintain balance; this is to help learn proper technique.

Sit-ups—Begin with your back flat against the floor, arms crossed over your chest, and your knees bent to ninety degrees. Bring your torso up until it touches your knee. Slowly bring your torso back down to the floor.

Flexed arm hang—Begin by hanging from a horizontal bar with arms flexed; then, with someone assisting, pull yourself up and lower yourself back down (as with pull-ups).

Note: Rather than focusing on the number of sets and repetitions for each exercise, focus on technique. Let the child look at this as "play" rather than organized exercise training.

Sample Advanced Training Session

Back squats (with light weight)—With a bar placed on the upper portion of your back (slightly above the shoulder blades but below the neck), keep your chin up and your back straight and taut as you descend into a squat position. Inhale as you descend. When your thighs are parallel to the floor, stop and begin your ascent slowly while exhaling.

Walking lunges (with no weight or with 1–2 pound dumbbells)—Hold a light dumbbell in each hand with your arms at your sides. Take a step forward with one leg so that your knee bends to a ninety-degree angle; at that moment, push forward with the back leg and come to a standing position. Then repeat the same motion with the other leg (to mimic a walking motion).

Training Age: Six to Ten Years

Training Tips

- Communicate with the child to see if he or she is still enjoying the training sessions and to check on how the child feels physically.
- Continue to introduce increasingly complex movements and add a few more exercises.
- Use light weights, bars, and dumbbells.
- Monitor motor skills, strength, balance, and posture.

- Keep coaching proper technique.

Sample Training Session

Back squats (with weight)—With a bar placed on the upper portion of your back (slightly above the shoulder blades but below the neck), keep your chin up and your back straight and taut as you descend into a squat position. Inhale as you descend. When your thighs are parallel to the floor, stop and begin your ascent slowly while exhaling.

Perform one set of twelve reps.

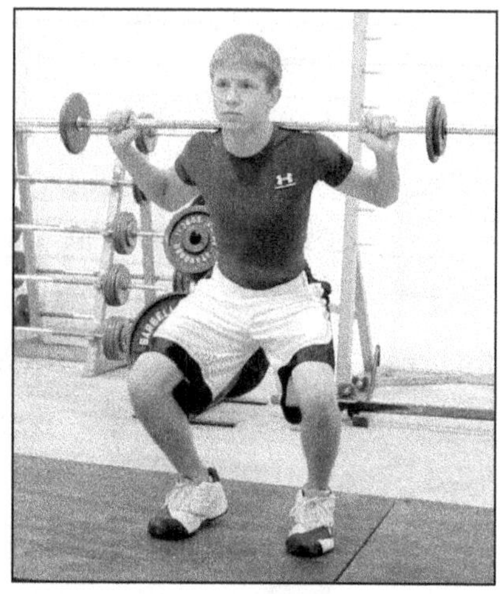

Back squat.

Leg curls—Lie face down on a leg curl machine. With your ankles underneath the pad, slowly curl your legs so that the ankles move toward your butt (inhale during this movement). Then slowly let the weight down as your ankles descend and your legs straighten out (exhale as you lower the weight).

Perform one set of twelve reps.

Bench press—To start, lie on the bench and grip the bar with your hands shoulder-width apart. Lift the bar off the rack and lower the weight slowly. The weight should just barely touch your chest before you push it back up (do not bounce the weight off your chest).

Perform one set of twelve reps.

Pull-ups—Use a wide, palms-out grip on a horizontal bar and pull yourself up to the point where your upper chest contacts the bar. Inhale on the way up and exhale as you descend slowly. During the movement, your legs should be bent slightly and you should avoid kicking to give yourself momentum (crossing your legs may help). If you can't do this alone, have a spotter assist you by holding your waist and giving you a slight push upward. This is a very difficult exercise for children (and even many adults) at first.

Perform one set of one to five reps.

Push-ups—Start with your hands shoulder-width apart and palms flat on the floor. With your arms extended to support your weight, keep your body straight, legs together, and toes firmly planted. Lower yourself in a steady and controlled manner until your chest touches the floor, then return to the upright position. Keep a firm and taut torso: don't let your back arch or your body sag at any point during the motion.

Perform one set of one to five reps.

Training Age: Ten to Twelve Years

Training Tips

- Keep up the communication with the child.
- Start introducing programs that are more advanced and training protocols that increase weight and intensity.
- Introduce the concept of sport-specific training and periodization. Periodization is a method of training that has caught on in the last ten years that involves focusing efforts on improving specific facets of fitness for predetermined periods of time. For example, a football player may follow a periodized plan. His off-season training regimen may start by focusing on adding new muscle mass and increasing strength. After a six- to eight-week period, he may then embark on a core strength–training regimen. The last cycle will then utilize the new mass and strength gains toward football-specific drills. Each phase will involve different exercises, volumes and speeds of training, repetition ranges, and rest periods. Since the body adapts so easily to types of training that are performed repeatedly, periodization is a great method for continually challenging the body and forcing new gains. (For more information, go to the website www.fitrex.com/periodization.shtml.)

- Make sure technique is continuing to progress.
- Keep it fun!

Sample Training Session

Walking lunges (with weight)—Hold a light dumbbell in each hand with your arms at your sides. Take a step forward with one leg so that your knee bends to a ninety-degree angle; at that moment, push forward with the back leg and come to a standing position. Then repeat the same motion with the other leg (to mimic a walking motion).

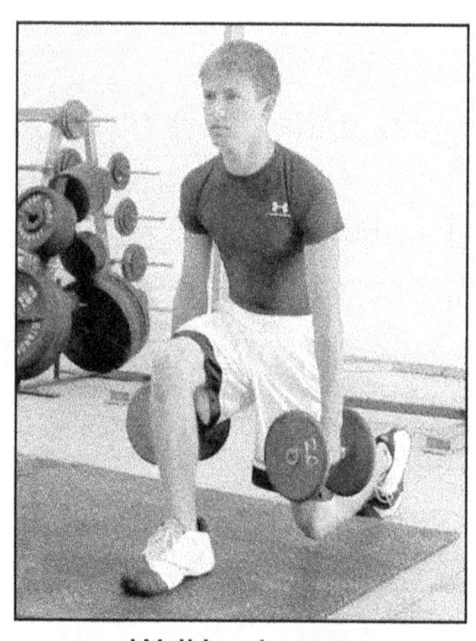

Walking lunge.

Back squats (with weight)—With a bar placed on the upper portion of your back (slightly above the shoulder blades but below the neck), keep your chin up and your back straight and taut as you descend into a squat position. Inhale as you descend. When your thighs are parallel to the floor, stop and begin your ascent slowly while exhaling.

Bench press—To start, lie on the bench and grip the bar with your hands shoulder-width apart. Lift the bar off the rack and lower the weight slowly. The weight should just barely touch your chest before you push it back up (do not bounce the weight off your chest).

Push-ups—Start with your hands shoulder-width apart and palms flat on the floor. With your arms extended to support your weight, keep your body straight, legs together, and toes firmly planted. Lower yourself in a steady and controlled manner until your chest touches the floor, then return to the upright position. Keep a firm and taut torso: don't let your back arch or your body sag at any point during the motion.

Shoulder press—You can use a straight barbell or light dumbbells for the shoulder press. Always maintain good posture when

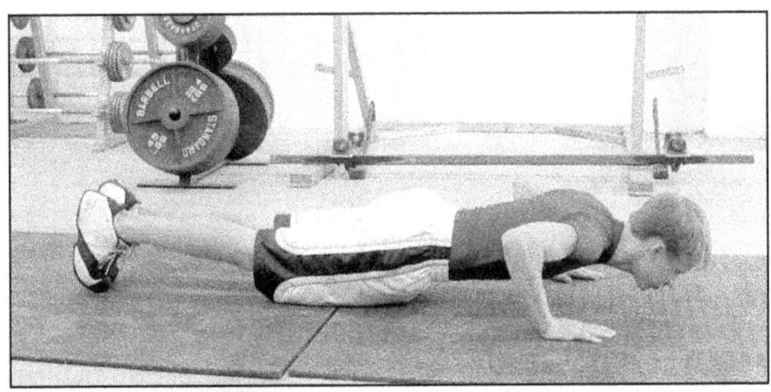

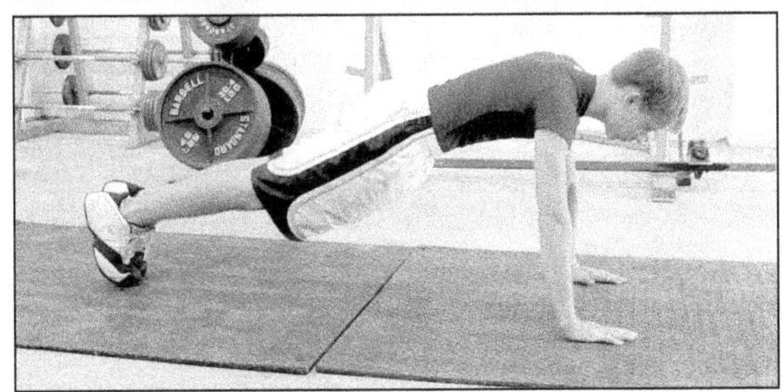

Push-ups are great for improving shoulder, chest, and core strength.

performing the movement. Keeping your back straight and your torso in a firm, taut position, start by holding the bar or dumbbells at shoulder level, with your palms facing out. Exhale during the upward motion as you push the weights straight up toward the ceiling, then inhale as you slowly lower the weights back to the starting position.

Pull-ups—Use a wide, palms-out grip on a horizontal bar and pull yourself up to the point where your upper chest contacts the bar. Inhale on the way up and exhale as you descend slowly. During the movement, your legs should be bent slightly and you should avoid kicking to give yourself momentum (crossing your legs may help). If you can't do this alone, have a spotter assist you by holding your waist and giving you a slight push upward. This is a very difficult exercise for children (and even many adults) at first.

Perform one to two sets of six to twelve repetitions per exercise.

Training Age: Thirteen and Older

Training Tips

- Continue to progress by increasing weight and intensity and working toward sport-specific training.
- Help to fine-tune technique.
- Develop programs using scientific progression (to make workouts harder over time) and periodization with the goal of peak performance.
- Focus on compound, multi-joint exercises.
- Learn from a certified strength-and-conditioning professional (see www.nsca-lift.org to find a trainer in your area).
- Use a spotter any time a teenager is lifting free weights.

Sample Training Session

Follow the sample training program for age ten to twelve years in the above section. Perform two to four sets of six to twelve repetitions per exercise.

FINAL THOUGHTS

Children can safely get involved in a resistance-training program that can help them in both daily, recreational activities and sports interests. If the training program is approached properly, your child can enjoy increased strength, prevent injuries, and improve his or her motor skills. Along with physical improvements, a child may also develop greater self-esteem and a lifetime commitment to fitness. Making sure your child progresses through the program safely will lead to a fun, exciting, and positive exercise experience.

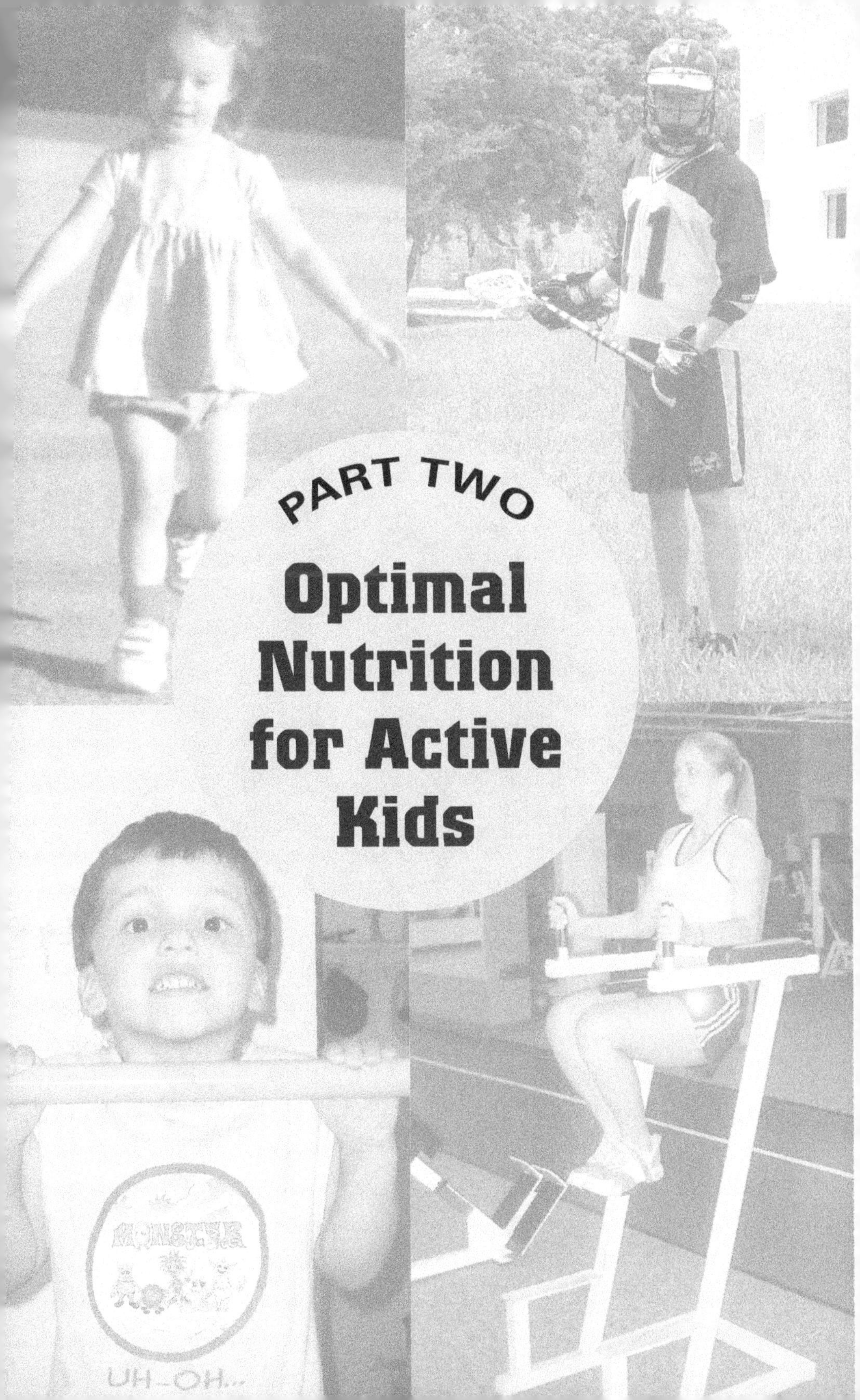

PART TWO
Optimal Nutrition for Active Kids

Basic Nutrition for Fit Kids

As a parent, you want to see your children succeed, prosper, and remain healthy throughout their lives. You sit down and help with their homework, play catch, and teach them the lessons of life so they don't make the same mistakes you did. Parents have a tremendous burden and responsibility in caring for their children. Instilling discipline is one of the hallmarks of raising a child and, interestingly, a lot of that discipline is introduced at the dinner table, isn't it? Well then, what better place to teach them some nutritional discipline as well?

Now, we are sure you're doing a fine job already. In hundreds of research studies spanning the last decade, there have been surprisingly few startling revelations concerning children and nutrition. Getting a child to eat their vegetables is no less important now than it was fifty years ago. But a parent's job rearing children is tougher than ever and, in the area of nutrition, it has become astoundingly difficult. Unlike fifty years ago, when dinner was at six o'clock sharp and the whole family ate together, we now deal with considerably more time constraints and outside influences that not only affect the way we live, but how we eat. We've become a society on the run.

The kids play sports after school and, if they want to compete with the Jones's kids, after practice they're in the gym getting stronger. They may also have band practice, the school play, a part-time job, and increasingly heavy loads of homework. This creates nutritional demands on the body, especially when sporadic and unhealthy eating is a habit. And then there's the current media obsession with thinness, which has undoubtedly affected the collective psyche of today's adolescents, especially impressionable young females. Throw in puberty, which is occurring at earlier ages than ever before, and parents end up with a monkey on their backs that just got bigger. Welcome to raising children, twenty-first-century style.

According to Patricia Ryan-Krause, R.N., the athletic adolescent is at a slightly higher risk for nutritional deficiencies because of increased energy needs.

In this chapter, we provide information to help you feed your kids right. This is critical not only for supporting their active lives now, but also for preventing ill health later in life. We'll explore the special nutritional requirements of active kids and give recommendations for healthy sources of protein, carbohydrates, and fats.

EAT RIGHT FOR AN ACTIVE LIFE

In the past, there was a preoccupation with simply meeting a child's nutritional needs (four food groups, vitamins, and so on), but now there's a major shift toward emphasizing the importance of childhood nutrition on health outcomes later in life. From eating habits themselves to preventing or encouraging disease processes, how your child eats today will have a striking impact on their health throughout adolescence and adulthood.

With the exception of early infancy, the human body grows the fastest during childhood and adolescence. For example, in just the early stages of puberty, children may gain up to 20 percent of their final adult height. This rapid growth makes proper nutrition a necessity and, without it, children may suffer harmful and irreversible effects on their growth and development.

Physical activity also takes its toll. The more kids exercise and participate in sports, the more calories and nutrients they need. They already require a substantial number of calories for proper growth, but sports activities place tremendous additional demands on the respiratory, cardiovascular, muscular, and skeletal systems. This is especially important today, when more kids at younger ages than ever before are participating in sports: there are 44.9 million children, ages six to eighteen, who play sports.[1] This places a special responsibility on parents, coaches, and the young athletes to understand the importance of high-quality nutrition.

MAXIMIZE GROWTH AND DEVELOPMENT IN CHILDREN AND ADOLESCENTS

Before we delve into the nuts and bolts of proper nutrition, we first need to define the age ranges for both children and adoles-

Young Athletes Differ from Adult Athletes

- Young athletes have a higher recommended protein intake (per body weight)
- Young athletes use relatively more fat as a fuel during exercise[2]
- The energy cost of walking and running is higher in young athletes
- During situations of dehydration, young athletes overheat faster[3]

Calcium Crisis?

Growing children and, in particular, adolescents may not be getting the calcium they need.

AGE	MEET CALCIUM NEEDS
Females 2–8 years	79%
Females 9–19 years	19%
Males 2–8 years	89%
Males 9–19 years	52%

Source: Health and Nutrition Examination Survey (Washington, D.C.: CDC, NCHS, 1988–1994).

cents so that we can address their unique needs. Specifically, we consider anyone under the age of ten or eleven as a growing child and from roughly ten to nineteen years of age as an adolescent. Adolescence is marked by puberty and a rapid growth rate, while growth during childhood is much slower. Nevertheless, even childhood presents challenges in obtaining nutritional requirements.

On average, children consume 1,700–1,800 calories per day and do pretty well in meeting their vitamin and mineral needs. That is, except for one mineral—calcium. It's an increasing concern that children and adolescents have experienced a decline in calcium intake in recent years. More than half of American children and adolescents fail to consume enough calcium, and they may even have higher needs in order to optimize bone health as they grow. According to a study from the *Journal of Internal Medicine,* "calcium intake during adolescence appears to affect skeletal calcium retention directly, and a calcium intake of up to 1,600 mg daily may be required."[4] Preferably, this should come from dietary staples such as milk and other dairy products because of their added health benefits.

In a fifteen-month study of calcium intake and exercise and

their effects on bone mineral status of girls sixteen to eighteen years old, scientists discovered that calcium supplementation (1,000 mg daily of calcium carbonate) increased mineral content in the lumbar spine, forearm, hip bone, and generally over the whole body.[5] The preservation of bone mineral content via calcium supplementation is one of several factors that affects bone mineralization later in life.[6]

Other than calcium needs, children usually have a good idea of how much food they need to maintain proper growth. But don't throw away those growth charts that your doctor uses. If your child is slipping behind what is considered normal height and weight for his or her age, an increase in caloric intake may be necessary. The current Recommended Dietary Allowance (RDA) for children seven to ten years old is 2,000 calories. Although this is a simple recommendation and may vary widely depending on a child's development, keep in mind that athletics may impose an additional need of 500–1,500 calories per day. That's why plotting your child's growth pattern and comparing it to established standards is probably the best way to ensure your child is eating enough (see www.cdc.gov/growthcharts). Overall, children should be encouraged to consume three meals a day plus nutrient-rich

Consequences of Inadequate Nutrition

- Short stature and delayed puberty
- Nutrient deficiencies and dehydration
- Menstrual irregularities
- Poor bone health
- Increased incidence of injuries
- Increased risk of developing eating disorders[7]

snacks. Of course, this is also assuming they are getting a fair amount of physical activity (video games don't count).

Meeting hydration needs is also critical for active kids. While appropriate nutrition ensures proper growth throughout their development, adequate hydration has immediate effects, such as preventing heat stress, heat stroke, and death. For anyone exercising, the primary mechanism for releasing body heat is through sweating. Unfortunately, kids can't sweat as much as adults and their bodies can overheat faster. This, of course, can be dangerous, so they need lots of water. Sports drinks are not necessary, although the flavor may help kids want to drink more. Just remember that thirst is not a good indicator of hydration needs; make sure kids consume 4–6 ounces of fluid every twenty to thirty minutes during exercise (see Chapter 6 for more information on hydration).

THE ENIGMATIC ADOLESCENT CONSUMER

Teenagers, probably as a result of peer pressure and a desire to be independent (how's that for a paradox?), have very unpredictable dietary habits. Some view food as the enemy and avoid it, either to stay thin or to compete successfully in sports such as wrestling and gymnastics. Many also skip breakfast and eat a lot of fast food and junk food. This can lead to a number of nutrient deficiencies.

For instance, one study found that competitive figure skaters, ages fourteen to sixteen, had intakes less than 50 percent of the RDA for calcium.[8] This is an unfortunate condition at a critical time in their lives for developing bone mass, especially because intense exercise in females can lead to amenorrhea (lack of menstruation) and thus a significant decrease in bone density, making proper calcium intake exceedingly important.

Exercise-induced amenorrhea, not an uncommon occurrence in females participating in ballet and gymnastics, can lead to a decline in estrogen, a highly beneficial hormone for bones. Research indicates that prolonged amenorrhea (two to three years)

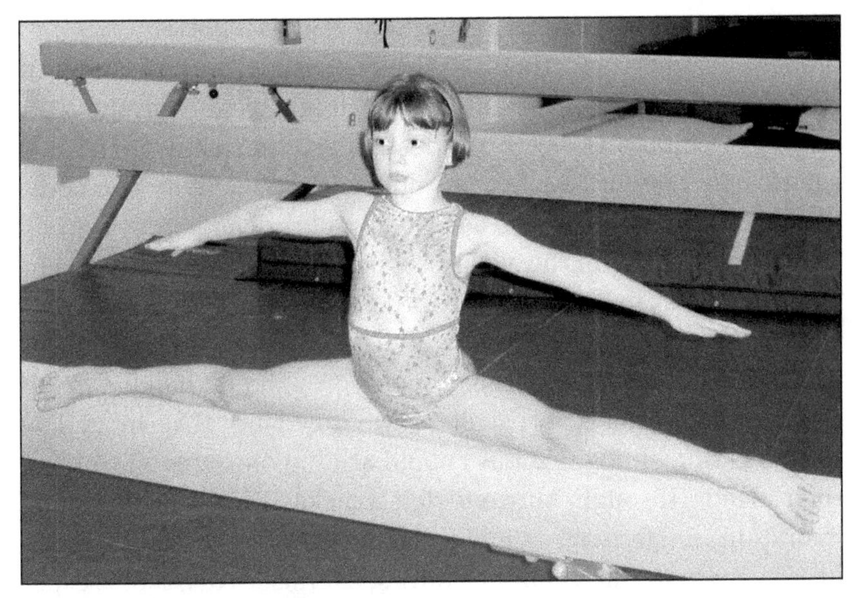

This female gymnast may require additional nutrients to maintain optimal health in her teenage years.

can cause irreversible bone loss. To combat this, teenagers need 1,200–1,500 mg of calcium daily to optimize bone health, and added protein, phosphorus, and vitamin D are also helpful for bone formation.

Iron is another crucial mineral for adolescents. Lack of iron limits exercise tolerance, while adequate amounts aid in proper growth and improve athletic performance.[9] Again, females are at risk of iron deficiency due to blood loss during menses, but males that train intensely may be deficient as well. Therefore, adolescents need about 15 mg of iron daily, with females possibly needing more, about 18 mg daily.[10] Athletes especially should be encouraged to eat iron-rich foods such as red meat, iron-fortified cereals, poultry, and green vegetables.

The rate of growth in adolescence is astounding, which means teenagers need calories, and lots of them, to ensure proper growth. Some teens have no problem: they love to eat everything in sight (which is only a problem if they don't exercise). The bigger concern is reserved for those who don't eat enough, especially if they are involved in sports that reward low body weight or a tiny figure (for example, wrestling, gymnastics, dance, and ice skating).

For males and females fifteen to eighteen years old, the RDA for energy intake is 3,000 calories per day for males and 2,200 calories per day for females. Of course, a lot of activity can boost this amount by 1,500–3,000 additional calories, and body size will also be a factor. Of the calories taken in, roughly 55 percent should come from carbohydrates, 30 percent from fat, and 15 percent from protein.

As in children, comparing a teen's growth and height/weight to standard norms is an excellent way to ensure that an adolescent is eating enough. Teens should also be encouraged to meet their needs through nutrient-rich snacks. Finally, concerning hydration, adolescents should consume 8–12 ounces of fluids every twenty to thirty minutes during exercise. This, too, is especially important in sports in which weight loss is sometimes encouraged. Adolescents need to consume enough fluids to maintain a clear, light-yellow, odorless urine.

RECOMMENDATIONS FOR IMPROVING PERFORMANCE IN SPORTS

For children and adolescents, there are a multitude of ways to use nutrition to improve performance in sporting activities. First and foremost, weigh kids on a regular basis to ensure continued growth. If they're not eating enough to grow, they're certainly not getting enough calories to thrive athletically. Encourage kids to drink plenty of fluids before, during, and after exercise, and have them consume additional carbohydrates about one hour before exercise or sporting events lasting longer than ninety minutes. Also, always encourage kids to eat breakfast and promote healthy snacking; this ensures adequate energy that will last throughout the day.

Do not restrict foods based on their fat content. Fat is a major source of energy, especially in children and adolescents, and provides most of the fuel for endurance events. Fat is also essential for hormone production, and sources of fat usually contain in-

Tips to Help Kids Eat a Healthy Diet

Some of these tips may apply to your situation while others may not. Take what is useful to you.

1 Don't make food an issue and don't put your kids on a "diet."

It amazes us that parents will put their children on restrictive diets, even if they're not fat. Don't force kids to eat a restricted list of foods and don't deny kids certain foods. Ultimately, your kids will make up their own minds about eating. They'll be quite capable of opening the refrigerator themselves and drinking soda, eating ice cream, and chowing down on pizza. Worse yet, they may end up hiding and hoarding foods because they're afraid you might disapprove of their food choices.

It's always best to show your child how to eat by example. Sure, it's okay for you as adults to have that occasional piece of chocolate (in fact, chocolate has some pretty healthy things in it, such as antioxidants), but eating a whole bag of chocolates is not the epitome of healthy eating. Also, your child will notice if you eat fibrous vegetables, lean sources of protein, and healthy carbohydrates. Your child will take note of your habits. In a sense, this book is as much about you, the parent, taking charge and leading by example. Being the passive bystander telling your child what to do may sometimes work, but only up to a point. It'll work better if you follow similar healthy habits.

Bottom line: Don't put your child on a restrictive diet and don't force him or her to eat certain foods. Tell your child what you believe is best (perhaps eat it yourself), offer the food to him or her, and eventually it will sink in. Your child will learn to make good food choices *most of the time.*

2 Perfection should never be the goal.

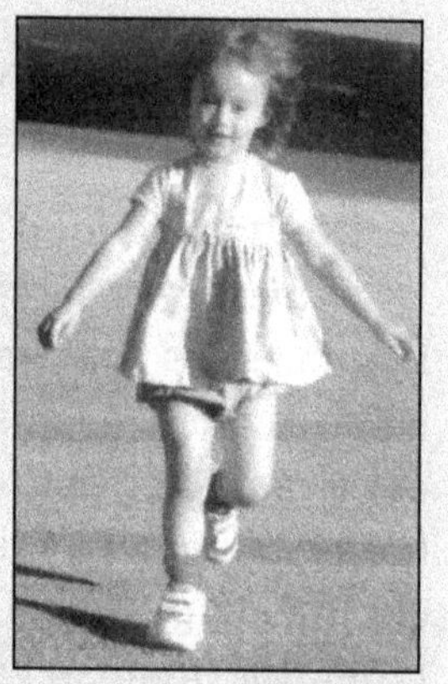

As long as your child eats well *most of the time* and is active *more often than not,* then that's good enough. If your child wants to train four hours a day doing gymnastics, karate, or any other exercise, let it be your child's decision. Of course, instill some common sense in your child if he or she thinks swimming for eight hours a day is healthy. Moderation still applies. But the parent who seeks perfection doesn't help the child: it will turn them off sports. First and foremost, sports or activity should be playful and fun. Don't deny your kids that pleasure.

Bottom line: The drive for perfection will make everyone crazy. Don't expect it from your child.

3 Limit processed foods.

We know your kids will eat whatever they want. Outside of putting a padlock on your fridge, your best bet is to refrain from buying items that are generally "empty calories." However, moderation is still the best approach. It's okay every once in a while for your kids to eat chips, cookies, cake, soda, and so on. This stuff is basically a lot of calories (sugar and fat) with little nutritive value. But let's face it, it tastes good! It's okay to "cheat" on your eating plan (more on "cheating" later), but limit these kinds of foods in your home.

Educate your children on how much better they will feel (vanity is clearly a major concern for many teenagers) if they eat unprocessed carbohydrates, lean protein, and vegetables. And they'll perform much better in sports (and academically) as well.

Just remember that if it doesn't occur naturally, then it's processed. For instance, white bread is processed, whereas broccoli, spinach, and lettuce are unprocessed since they are natural. Ever heard of a ketchup tree? A mayonnaise shrub? A cereal bush? These are processed foods that don't occur in nature. When in doubt, eat unprocessed foods!

Bottom line: Eating well most of the time is the goal.

4 Supplement your child's eating, when it is necessary. We know the word *supplements* often denotes energy-boosting pills and protein powders that bodybuilders consume to get larger muscles. First of all, there is nothing magical about the majority of supplements on the market. For instance, if you take a multivitamin, you're taking a supplement. Common foods such as bread, milk, and orange juice are fortified with various vitamins and minerals (like calcium), so you're eating "supplements" whether you are aware of it or not.

The fact is that most of us do not eat perfectly. Having your child take a multivitamin won't replace proper eating habits, but at least he or she will get the nutrients that may otherwise be missing from the diet. However, supplementation should always be a second choice—eating the right foods is clearly the primary goal. If you can get your child to eat a dinner that consists of a cup of broccoli, a cup of brown rice, and baked skinless chicken, congratulations! But if he or she would rather eat chips and a soda, then multivitamin supplementation is probably needed.

What about other supplements such as protein powders, energy bars, or protein shakes? Again, it's best to encourage your child to get their protein from unprocessed foods such as chicken, turkey, lean cuts of beef, and fish. But if given the choice between an unhealthy snack laden with fat and sugar or a protein shake, go with the shake. For instance, one of the popular brands of protein shakes contains 40 grams of protein (mainly milk protein), 15 grams of carbohydrates, and 3 grams of fat for a grand total of 240 calories. Contrast that with a one-patty hamburger with condiments, large fries, and a cola, which adds up to 1,190 calories (19 grams of protein, 199 grams of carbohydrates, and 35 grams of fat). If your child consistently chooses the burgers and fries, he or she will enter the ranks of the fat and unfit. It certainly would be helpful, once in a while, if the protein shake were chosen over the fast food.

5 Cheating is a must!

You've taught your child that cheating is wrong, but when it comes to diet and exercise, cheating is a fundamental part of the program! What we mean is that it's okay, every once in a while, to let your child eat junk food. And it's okay if your child doesn't want to exercise every day. Perfection isn't the goal; maintaining healthy habits that will carry into adulthood is.

So, if you find your kid snacking on a glazed donut, let him enjoy it. Of course, if you see him eating like this every day, then it's time to put the brakes on the sugar. The whole point of cheating is to give your body and mind a break from what can often become a routine. As important as exercise and good eating is for your body, sometimes you just want to escape it all. Being lazy and eating junk food is occasionally warranted.

So, how often should cheating be allowed? If you can get your child to eat well 60 to 70 percent of the time, that's great. With exercise, as long as he or she is doing some sort of activity about three times per week, then that's about right. Anything less than that requires friendly encouragement from you to your child to get off the couch and go out and play!

creased levels of important nutrients such as iron, protein, and calcium. Stay away from junk foods and sources high in saturated fats (these should make up no more than 10 percent of total calories). Also, cholesterol should not exceed 300 mg per day.

Dealing with children and nutrition can be an everyday ordeal. Although it's easier to just heat up a microwave dinner, maintaining proper nutrition in children is simply a process, not unlike promoting the right study habits. It's work, but your child may be rewarded with higher athletic skills and exceptional health that will last a lifetime.

PROTEIN POWER

Protein is a macronutrient that really hasn't gotten a fair shake. Myths abound about protein: it's bad for your kidneys, it'll dehydrate you, it'll make your bones brittle. Too much protein is the proverbial evil of the macronutrient world (fat may be a close second). But all these beliefs are unfounded, particularly when it comes to the growing, active child. Let's examine why protein is so important for children and teenagers who participate in sports. And then we'll take the three myths and give you the real story.

The word *protein* is derived from the Greek word meaning "of prime importance." It's important because enzymes, antibodies, cell membranes, muscle, organs, and an array of other body parts are comprised of protein. Besides water, your body is mainly protein.

The building blocks of protein are amino acids. If you string a bunch of amino acids together, you basically have a protein. That is why milk protein can be distinguished from egg protein by looking at amino acid composition, as well as the rate at which the proteins are digested. You will see that certain proteins are "fast absorbing" while others are "slow absorbing."

Essential amino acids are those amino acids that you need to eat because your body doesn't normally make them. The main reason for consuming dietary protein is to provide the essential amino acids your body needs. Animal proteins have all of the essential amino acids.

Eggs, milk, and meat contain all the essential amino acids; if you eat these foods, you'll meet your body's protein needs. On the other hand, if you eat nonanimal sources, you'll need to combine certain foods (such as beans and rice) to get all of the essential amino acids. The reason for this is that certain grains and vegetables are too low in some amino acids. To make up for that low level, you need to combine them with foods containing high levels of the lacking amino acid—hence, the popular beans and rice combo. The only source of plant protein that contains all the essential amino acids is soy. So, if you're a strict vegetarian, you should combine your foods, and eat soy protein.

Essential amino acids are those amino acids that you need to eat because your body doesn't normally make them. Animal proteins have all of the essential amino acids.

Protein is essential for normal health, growth, and development of young athletes. Without adequate protein, the child's development is impaired and athletic performance suffers. Kids who exercise need more protein than their couch-potato counterparts. But unlike adults, kids are still growing. So if you combine the energy costs of normal growth with the energy costs of exercise, young kids likely have a greater need for protein (for a given body weight) than adults.

How Much Protein Should a Young Athlete Consume?

According to the latest standards for Recommended Dietary Allowances (RDAs), the amount of protein needed by young kids may exceed that of adults. The current adult RDA for protein is 0.8 grams of protein daily per *kilogram* of body weight (0.36 grams of protein per pound of body weight). However, that level is too low for adults who exercise. Thus, it makes sense that the recommendations for active children are also too low. And for kids who play multiple sports, the RDA is completely inadequate.

Children need a greater protein intake in order to satisfy the growth requirements of their bodies.[11] Additionally, children use more energy to move their bodies; that is, for a given body weight, a child requires more calories to move than an adult does. For healthy adults who participate in endurance or weight-training exercises, protein needs are approximately 0.6 to 0.9 grams of protein per *pound* of body weight (1.3 to 2.0 grams of protein per kilogram of body weight). It would seem reasonable that the protein needs of a child, and in particular of a growing teenager who is exercising, would be on the higher end of that spectrum. Thus, for a fifteen-year-old boy who weighs 150 pounds and is participating in multiple sports, consuming roughly 135 grams of protein daily is a must.

For simplicity's sake, a lot of athletes try to consume 1 gram of protein per *pound* of body weight. Thus, for a 150-pound individual, that would translate into 150 grams of protein daily.

Protein Sources

There are a multitude of high-quality proteins to choose from: milk protein (which is mainly casein and whey), soy, meats, fish, and egg whites are all wonderful protein sources. Basically, the protein you eat should provide the entire complement of essential amino acids. The essential amino acids include the branched-chain amino acids (valine, leucine, isoleucine), lysine, methionine, phenylalanine, threonine, histidine, and tryptophan. Incomplete proteins, such as from peanuts, do not contain all the essential amino acids.

Animal proteins carry the entire complement of amino acids, so if you are trying to gain weight for the football team, complete proteins should be an important part of your eating regimen. Alternatively, if you don't like eating animal products for whatever reason, you could consume more plant foods to make up for the poor quality of most plant proteins (except soy). For example, a slice of whole-wheat bread contains less than 2 grams of protein, and the quality of this protein is less than a third of that of egg or milk protein. So, you'd have to eat approximately 146 slices of bread to meet the requirements of a young male who regularly exercises. Now, that's a lot of white bread! And that doesn't take into account that white bread is a processed carbohydrate, which is not a very good food choice.

Preferred protein sources include fish, lean meat, eggs (or egg whites), or some form of meal-replacement powder that contains whey, soy, or casein protein.

Whey and Casein

"Little Miss Muffet sat on a tuffet eating her curds and whey . . ." Do you remember that nursery rhyme? Well, the curds (casein) and whey are both high-quality proteins derived from milk. You can consume whey if you drink a lot of milk (but even that's mostly casein) or if you consume a meal-replacement powder. Whey is an excellent protein source and there are many studies showing that whey might improve body composition and health.

Casein, the main protein in milk, is also an excellent protein source. It is absorbed very slowly into your bloodstream, so you can get sustained levels of amino acids in your blood. This is important because these amino acids go into muscle fibers and help them repair and regenerate. When you eat whey protein, you'll experience a quick rise in blood levels of amino acids, followed by a steady decline. On the other hand, if you consume casein protein, you'll get a slow and sustained increase in blood amino acids over several hours. By combining the two proteins, you get the best of both worlds: a quick rise in amino acid levels from the whey and a slower increase in blood amino acids from the casein. This occurs because whey protein empties quickly from the stomach, while casein clots in the stomach and tends to be absorbed much slower.

Why is it important to keep blood amino acid levels high? Having this constant pool of amino acids will allow you to make new protein (such as muscle fibers). It will also help in the repair of damaged muscle tissue resulting from intense exercise. So, consume lots of milk or one of an assortment of meal-replacement powders that contain both proteins.

Soy

Soy offers a variety of benefits similar to those provided by whey. For instance, there is some evidence that soy has anticarcinogenic effects and may also improve body composition.[12] If you're a vegetarian, soy is perhaps your best protein option, because it contains all of the essential amino acids.

The Maligned Egg

Eggs are much maligned, accused of promoting heart disease and contributing to expanding waistlines. So, should your child eat whole eggs? If you want a high-quality protein, eggs should be included (egg white and yolk). Eggs have a full complement of the essential amino acids—a complete protein. In addition, eggs are a rich source of thiamine, riboflavin, pantothenic acid, folic acid, vitamin B_{12}, biotin, vitamins D and E, and phosphorus.

A study from the University of Tennessee Health Science Center concluded that there was no association between egg consumption (one or more eggs daily) and the risk of coronary heart disease in nondiabetic men and women.[13] Clearly, eggs are not as harmful as many "experts" suggest. It's just nonsense that eating one egg a day is bad for your heart; it is a claim unsupported by science. Thus, we reiterate that your child can consume eggs regularly without harm.

Egg Facts *(one large whole egg)*

• Calories: 77 • Protein: 6.3 grams

• Carbohydrates: 0.6 grams • Fat: 5.3 grams

Fish

What makes fish so great as a protein source is its fat content: you will not find a better source of healthy fats than the kind found in fish (like salmon). Of course, the protein in fish is complete and good for you, but the added benefit of fish is that it contains two major polyunsaturated fats: eicosapentaenoic acid (EPA) and docosahexaenoic acid (DHA), both omega-3 fats. Studies show that Greenland Eskimos, who eat lots of fish, have a lower incidence of heart disease.[14] The beneficial effects of EPA and DHA are numerous, including an anti-inflammatory role, which may help injured muscles recover from intense exercise.[15]

Taking some fish-oil supplements or, better yet, eating lots of fish will expedite the postexercise recovery process.

Chicken, Turkey, Beef, and Pork

Take the skin off chicken or turkey and you've got a fairly lean and healthy source of protein. What would athletes do if they couldn't eat white-meat chicken breast? A bodybuilder's favorite meal often includes grilled skinless chicken breast, a cup of broccoli, and a small serving of brown rice. Chicken and turkey are great, low-fat sources of protein that certainly taste better than a protein powder shake. But unlike whey or soy, chicken meat does not confer any special health benefits; the same is true of beef and pork. They are great sources of protein, but many cuts of meat are loaded with saturated fat. So, go easy on the beef and pork, but don't completely eliminate these foods for the family; let your child indulge once in awhile.

When Should Athletes Eat Protein?

Kids who exercise need to eat protein frequently throughout the day to ensure that they have amino acids readily available for making extra muscle protein, or just to aid in postexercise recovery. Research has shown that muscle protein synthesis (the building-up process) was increased at four hours and twenty-four hours after exercise, but returned to pre-exercise levels after

Is Excess Protein Bad for Your Kids?

How often have you heard rumors of the dangers of excessive protein consumption? A book on sports nutrition discusses the potential dangers of excess protein and you're left to wonder what's the truth of the matter. Well, as is often the case, many "experts" are misinformed. There is *no* evidence that a high protein intake is harmful to normal, healthy individuals. Certainly, consuming twice the RDA (1.6 grams of protein daily per kilogram of body weight) has no known ill effects. Unless your liver or kidneys are failing, then it's really just a phantom health issue that is perpetually promulgated by those who should know better. Two recent studies reported in *The American Journal of Clinical Nutrition* will hopefully lay to rest the notion that excess protein is dangerous. It turns out that high protein intakes may actually be healthy.

In a study from the University of Copenhagen in Denmark, scientists compared the effects of dietary soy versus casein protein on lipoprotein-a, or Lp(a), concentrations in nine healthy men. High levels of blood Lp(a) are associated with heart disease. Interestingly, diets low in saturated fat (animal fat) and cholesterol have no effect on Lp(a) levels. The role of dietary proteins on Lp(a) levels is not entirely known, but this study shed light on the healthy effects of protein, particularly casein. These men consumed three types of diets in a randomized order for thirty days each: a self-selected diet, a soy-protein diet, and a casein-protein diet. At the end of the study, the casein-protein diet produced a dramatic drop in Lp(a) levels, while the soy-protein and self-selected diets had no effect. Thus, casein protein (one of the main proteins in various meal-replacement powders) may decrease cardiovascular risk.[16]

A study from Johns Hopkins University in Baltimore looked at the effects of protein consumption on blood concentrations of homocysteine (Hcy). Elevated levels of Hcy have been shown to increase the risk of cardiovascular disease, independent of any other coronary risk factors. The study involved 260 retired schoolteachers. Researchers found that as protein intake increased, total Hcy concentration in the blood decreased. Those who ate 36–48 grams of protein per day had Hcy levels that were 30 percent higher than those who consumed up to 94 grams of protein per day. This amount of protein per day is not high by bodybuilding standards; it is uncertain if further increases in protein result in additional reductions in Hcy.[17]

These studies indicate that protein intake is not harmful and instead may be good for you. Casein protein, in particular, seems to have the most health benefits. While these studies were performed on adults, you may conclude that, even in growing kids and teenagers, there is no evidence that eating twice the RDA for protein is harmful. Besides, if you have a child who is both growing and exercising, it would seem sensible that his or her protein needs supersede those of an adult.

thirty-six hours.[18] So, there is a one- to two-day window of time to take advantage of the fact that the body is primed for nutrient uptake. What it needs most is high-quality protein.

For example, if your kids exercise at noon, assume that you'll need to feed their muscles all day while they are awake, all through the night while asleep, and then again in the early morning in order to meet their protein needs after a single session of exercise! When should they eat protein? As a general rule, protein should be eaten at breakfast, lunch, and dinner. And, this is important, have them eat a protein-containing snack between breakfast and lunch and again between lunch and dinner.

Also, right after they finish exercising, make sure they consume a small meal that contains twice as many carbohydrates as protein, with a touch of fat. The carbohydrates will ensure that muscle glycogen stores are replenished, and the protein is needed for repairing damaged muscle fibers; fat is to replenish intramuscular fat deposits, which are used for energy during subsequent exercise bouts.

In a nutshell, protein is needed for the normal recovery process after exercise, as well as for adding extra muscle mass. The paltry amount recommended in the government's RDA will not meet the needs of active individuals. In fact, eating at least twice the RDA is necessary. The best proteins to eat are eggs, milk, whey, casein, soy, and meats (beef, fish, chicken, turkey), while most vegetable protein sources are inferior. Some of these proteins, particularly whey and soy, as well as the fat in fish, offer health benefits to the heart and immune system. When your kids eat is as important as what they eat: small frequent meals are imperative, and each meal should contain a high-quality protein with a starchy, unprocessed carbohydrate and a fibrous vegetable.

CARBOHYDRATES—THE BODY'S MAIN FUEL

Carbohydrates are the single most frequently consumed food in the world and carbohydrate-containing foods are often the best tasting as well. Cakes, cookies, fudge, chocolates . . . the list goes on. We love our carbs and our kids love them as well.

The term *carbohydrate* refers to all sugars, but as with anything else in nutrition, nothing is ever that simple. The sugar we're most familiar with is table sugar or sucrose, but there is also fruit sugar (fructose) and milk sugar (lactose). Ultimately, whatever form of carbohydrate you consume eventually is converted to glucose (blood sugar) or glycogen (the form in which your body stores carbohydrates), primarily in the liver and skeletal muscles.

Nutritionists generally classify carbohydrates based on the

number of sugar molecules that are linked together: monosaccharides, disaccharides, and polysaccharides.

- A *monosaccharide* has just one sugar molecule (*mono* means one). The monosaccharides that are nutritionally important include fructose (fruit sugar) and glucose. Not all simple sugars or monosaccharides are treated the same by the body. For instance, fructose is primarily converted to glucose by the liver. Interestingly, fructose tends to promote fat synthesis (or gain) more so than other sugars. Glucose (or its stored form, glycogen) is the form of sugar that is most important for the body's chemical reactions needed for exercise.
- Table sugar or sucrose is a *disaccharide*—that is, two sugars put together: a glucose and a fructose molecule. This sugar is the most commonly consumed simple sugar. Lactose is another disaccharide, glucose plus galactose, and is found in milk. Lactose is the least sweet form of sugar (fructose is the sweetest). The problem with lactose, however, is that many people have an intolerance to it, which causes stomach and intestinal problems (gas, stomachaches).
- *Polysaccharides* or complex carbohydrates include starches and fiber, the most nutrient-dense carbohydrates you can eat (whole-grain breads, pastas, brown rice, wheat, beans, peas, potatoes, and roots).

Plant starches are the most important carbohydrate component of your diet. These are the carbohydrates you should emphasize, whereas simple sugars are the ones to de-emphasize. An easy way to remember this is to eat the carbohydrates that are in the produce section of the grocery store, mainly fresh fruit and vegetables. If you can get your kid to eat *one serving* of these each day, that is, in and of itself, a major victory.

The Glycemic Index

The glycemic index is a measure of how much blood sugar or glu-

Glycemic Index (GI) Ratings of Common Foods

The values for the glycemic index are based on the notion that the consumption of glucose produces the highest GI and is given the arbitrary designation of 100. Thus, a food with a GI rating of 50 has half the glucose response of pure glucose.

Low GI Rating (below 50):	***Moderate GI Rating (50–75):***	***High GI Rating (over 75):***
Apples	Balance Bar	Cakes
Butter	Bananas	Carrots
Fructose	Brown rice	Cookies
Grapes	Corn	Cornflakes
Lentils	Mixed-grain breads	Glucose
Low-carbohydrate bars (Atkins Advantage bar)	Oatmeal	High-carbohydrate bars, such as PowerBar*
Meats	Potato chips	Potatoes
Milk	Sucrose (table sugar)	Pretzels
Navy beans	Sweet potatoes	Raisins
Oranges	White pasta	Saltine crackers
Peanut butter		Shredded wheat
Peanuts		White bread
Pinto beans		White rice
Soy		
Spaghetti, protein-enriched		
Split peas		

**The PowerBar produces a greater glycemic and insulin response than white bread[19])*

So you can see that table sugar has a lower glycemic-index rating than white bread, white rice, carrots, potatoes, and so on. Try to choose foods that have a low GI

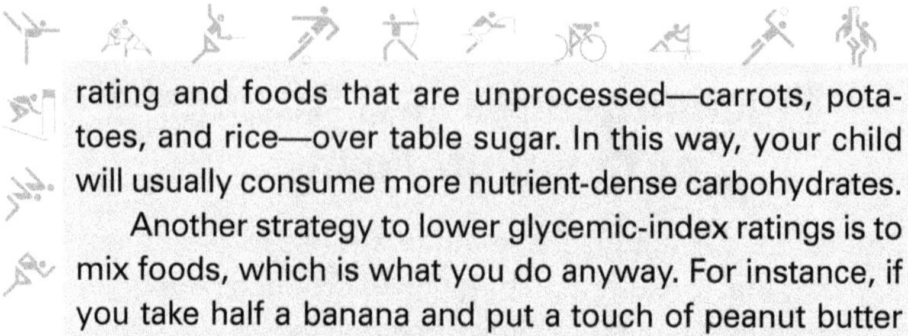

rating and foods that are unprocessed—carrots, potatoes, and rice—over table sugar. In this way, your child will usually consume more nutrient-dense carbohydrates.

Another strategy to lower glycemic-index ratings is to mix foods, which is what you do anyway. For instance, if you take half a banana and put a touch of peanut butter on it, it'll make the combination a lower glycemic food choice and a healthy one as well. Also, protein and fat in a meal will slow down the absorption of carbohydrates.

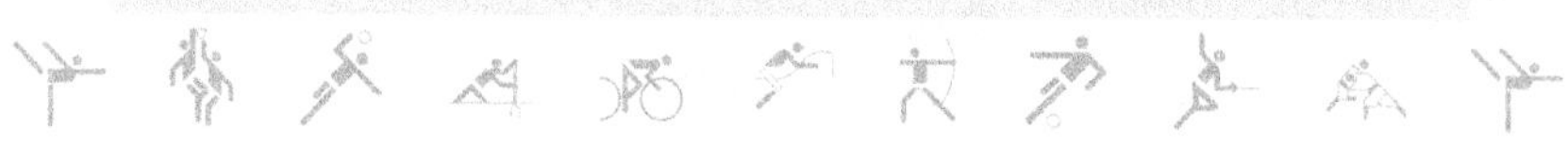

cose rises in a given period of time after ingesting 50 grams of a particular carbohydrate. High-glycemic carbohydrates include potatoes, raisins, white rice, and carrots; low-glycemic carbohydrates include fructose, milk products, yogurt, peas, and beans. Eating high-glycemic carbohydrates results in an oversecretion of insulin, which may predispose you to depositing fat and increase your risk for various diseases.

The glycemic index can provide some very important information for choosing healthy foods, but it isn't the only factor in deciding which foods are best for your child. For instance, it is generally accepted that it is best to eat low-glycemic carbohydrates instead of the high-glycemic variety because they are healthier. And for the most part, that is correct: beans, brown rice, and legumes are great sources of carbohydrates, vitamins, minerals, and some protein as well. But on the flip side, you have some high-glycemic carbohydrates, such as carrots and potatoes, that are also wholesome foods. Interestingly, table sugar has a lower glycemic index than a similar serving of carrots or potatoes. So, are we suggesting you consume table sugar instead of carrots or potatoes? Absolutely not. In fact, if you look at the lists of foods under "Glycemic Index (GI) Ratings of Common Foods," you'll see that some unprocessed, nutrient-dense carbohydrates have a higher glycemic index than simple, nutrient-sparse sugars.

Carbohydrates for the Young Athlete

Most young athletes expend energy both from exercise and from the requirements of a growing body, so their bodies have a heightened need for replenishment. Regardless of the age of the athlete, carbohydrates and fat are the main fuel sources that the body uses for energy. Some experts recommend that at least 55 percent of the caloric intake come from carbohydrates. Whether or not this is the "ideal" level of carbohydrates isn't really known. Instead of sticking to a percentage, emphasize the unprocessed carbohydrates over the processed ones (most breads, pastas, cookies, candy, cakes, and so on). How do you tell the difference? Well if it's in a package or it has a label, then it is processed; exceptions include various kinds of beans that you can buy in a can, which are good carbohydrates. As a general rule, if it's in a box, it isn't natural.

High Glycemic Foods and the Heart

In a study from the *American Journal of Clinical Nutrition,* scientists found that dietary glycemic load was directly associated with the risk of heart disease. Those who consumed the most high-glycemic carbohydrates had a higher risk of heart disease. Researchers concluded that "the current low-fat, high-carbohydrate diet recommended in the United States may not be optimal for the prevention of coronary heart disease and could actually increase the risk in individuals with high degrees of insulin resistance and glucose tolerance."[20]

Even though this study was done with adults, it seems reasonable that if your child starts eating lots of high-glycemic carbohydrates now, it may increase his or her risk for heart disease as an adult.

You've probably heard the term *carbohydrate loading* (or "carb loading" for short)—this refers to a technique that marathon runners sometimes use. In essence, it involves eating a very large volume of carbohydrates for a couple days prior to running a race. What this does is fill up your muscles' stores of glycogen (the stored form of carbohydrate). Increasing your glycogen, theoretically, should give your muscles more energy to burn. As promising as this technique might be, it is not needed for young kids participating in regular activities. Even if a child plays all day and expends a lot of energy, his or her normal carbohydrate intake should adequately replace the used stores of muscle glycogen.

FATS—THE GOOD AND THE BAD

Of the major macronutrients (carbohydrates, protein, fat), fat has perhaps the worst reputation. Fat has 9 calories per gram, which is more than twice the calories of a protein or carbohydrate. So, eating fat must make you fat, right? And if that's the case, then we need to protect our kids from too much of it. It's not that simple.

You've probably heard of the so-called Mediterranean diet—a diet based on the eating patterns of Greece and Southern Italy that is rich in fruits, vegetables, grains, and omega-3 fatty acids, but low in meat and saturated fats. Well, about 40 percent of the dietary calories in the Mediterranean diet come from fat—that's more than in the average American's diet. If fat is bad for you, then people who eat the Mediterranean diet must have higher disease rates and other problems, right? In a word, no: people on this diet are healthy.

The important thing to remember is the *kind* of fat consumed. The foundation of the Mediterranean diet is consuming high levels of olive oil. Olive oil, perhaps the healthiest of all oils, is a monounsaturated fat that is a good source of antioxidants, nutrients that can protect the body from the damaging effects of free radicals (metabolic byproducts that can harm your cells). Olive oil and monounsaturated fats in general are heart healthy and can decrease your risk of cardiovascular disease.

We also know that monounsaturated fats are less likely to be stored in the body as fat. You know when you pinch an inch around your waist? Well, this kind of fat is less apt to end up there, unlike the kinds of fat in margarine (trans fats) or in a fatty cut of meat (saturated fat).

Your child needs to eat healthy fats. Having a child on a low-fat diet is complete nonsense: it's bad for their health and will likely stunt their growth. Instead, promote plant fats (such as olive oil) and fish fats in your child's diet. Eating burgers and fries will provide lots of fat, but it's mainly saturated fat; and if your child has the choice, he or she will probably pick the burgers and fries. So, encourage your child to eat fish at least once a week.

Types of Fat

Fats are classified as saturated and unsaturated. Saturated fats are solid at room temperature and include beef fat, butter, margarine, and cream cheese. These are the fats that you should try to limit, but don't eliminate them from your kid's diet.

The unsaturated fats, which are liquid at room temperature, are either monounsaturated or polyunsaturated, depending on their chemical structure. Monounsaturated fats have one "double bond" within the fat molecule, while polyunsaturated fats have more than one double bond. Examples of monounsaturated fats are olive oil, almond oil, canola oil, and peanut oil. Of course, if you eat nuts or olives, you'll be getting good amounts of these healthy fats as well. Polyunsaturated fats include safflower oil, corn oil, and sunflower oil.

As we mentioned earlier, the two polyunsaturated fats eicosapentaenoic acid (EPA) and docosahexaenoic acid (DHA) are particularly healthy. In fact, these omega-3 fats are downright great for you! They are found in cold-water fish, such as tuna, herring, salmon, sardines, and mackerel. If your child doesn't like fish, then he or she is missing out on some of the healthiest fats. Regular consumption of fish (and fish oils) can reduce the risk of heart disease. Also, fish fat is anti-inflammatory, which may be beneficial for healing injured or sore muscles, allowing your child to recover more quickly from the soccer match or swimming practice. Again, if you can get your child to eat fish once every week, it would be wonderful for their health.

Watch Out for Partially Hydrogenated Oil

Pick up a jar of real peanut butter, the kind with nothing added: it has a slightly rough texture to it and doesn't spread so easily. But processed peanut butter spreads nice and smoothly. Why? Processed peanut butter contains partially hydrogenated oil, what nutritionists call trans fats. And they are bad for your health. For instance, a study from the Netherlands found that consuming trans fats decreased HDL levels in the blood (a drop in HDL levels increases the potential risk of heart disease).[21] The problem is that some of your child's favorite foods probably have lots of trans fats: cookies, crackers, jellies, ice cream. Read the labels of these processed foods and you'll see they contain partially hydrogenated fat. Chemically modifying these fats by adding hydrogen molecules to them makes the fat smoother, with a better texture. That's why processed peanut butter spreads so easily.

While it's virtually impossible to eliminate trans fats completely because they are in nearly all processed foods, eating should be about healthy percentages. As long as you have your child pick the right foods most of the time, then don't worry so much about occasional lapses.

Good Sources of Fat

- Almonds
- Avocados
- Cashews
- Fish (especially cold-water fish like salmon, tuna, and herring)

- Non-processed vegetable oils
- Nuts (in general)
- Olive oil or olives
- Peanut butter or peanuts

Fats to Limit

- Any foods with "partially hydrogenated" on the label
- Chicken/turkey skin
- Fats from beef and pork
- Margarine
- Whole milk

Healthy Meals and Snacks

The previous chapter looked at the basics of healthy eating for active kids. Now, on a practical level, you need to find convenient foods that will give your kids the nutrition they need *and* fit your hectic schedule. There are many ways to fuel your kids' bodies so that they maintain energy levels throughout the day. You probably don't have time to count calories or grams of carbohydrates and fat. Instead, we suggest that you provide your child with various food choices, both foods to emphasize and foods to limit. Many of the foods that you emphasize may not be on your child's list of top foods, and the foods you limit may be among their favorites. But part of teaching children proper nutrition is presenting them with good and not-so-good choices. Ultimately, they will learn what foods serve them best. Besides, you can't force your child to eat good foods. It's like the old proverb: Catch a fish for someone and you feed him for a day, but if you teach him to fish, you feed him for life. Teach your child to "fish" for healthy foods.

THREE HEALTHY MEAL PLANS

While it's helpful to have a list of good and bad foods, here we also provide several healthy meals you can give your growing child or teenager. They emphasize quality protein, unprocessed carbohydrates, and healthy fats.

Foods to Emphasize

Proteins:

Eggs

Fish (broiled, baked, but not fried)

Lean beef (high in iron and zinc)

Milk protein (whey and casein; found mainly in protein powders and ready-to-drink protein shakes)

Skim/1% milk

Skinless chicken/turkey breast

Soy

Tuna

Carbohydrates:

Brown rice

Dry beans

Fruits, such as:
- apples
- bananas
- blueberries
- peaches
- pears
- strawberries

Green vegetables

Whole-grain bread

Whole oatmeal

Yams, sweet potatoes

Fat:

Almonds

Cashews

Fish oils (DHA and EPA)

Macadamia nuts

Peanut butter (unprocessed)

Peanuts

Walnuts

Foods to Limit

Proteins:

Beef (fatty cuts, such as ground beef)

Cold cuts/lunch meats

Fried foods

Hot dogs

Carbohydrates:

Anything with lots of sugar

Boxed cereals (choose high-fiber, natural cereals; others are mainly sugar)

Cakes

Candy

Cookies

Crackers (saltine)

Desserts

Pastries

Pizza

Sodas with sugar

White bread

White rice

Fats:

Butter

Fat from cold cuts, fatty meats

Fat from fried foods

Hydrogenated oils or trans fats (in many processed, packaged foods)

Ice cream

Margarine

DAY ONE

Breakfast: 2-egg omelet filled with 1 slice of turkey and 1 slice of cheese; $1/_2$ cup of oatmeal; 1 cup of 1% milk

Snack: Yogurt (1 serving)

Lunch: Chicken sandwich on whole-wheat bread with lettuce, tomato slices, and mustard; 1 small banana; 12 ounces of water

Dinner: Barbecued chicken (1–2 breasts), 1 cup of green vegetables (such as broccoli or spinach), 1 cup of cooked brown rice; 12 ounces of water

Snack: 1 cup of 1% milk

DAY TWO

Breakfast: 2 pancakes made from oat flour; 1 slice of ham; $1/_2$ banana; 1 cup of 1% milk

Snack: Apple or banana with 1 teaspoon of peanut butter

Lunch: Chicken fajitas with guacamole and salsa; 12 ounces of water

Dinner: 1 cup of cooked spaghetti, with $1/_4$ pound of lean ground beef and marinara sauce; $1/_2$ cup of broccoli on the side; 12 ounces of water

Snack: Yogurt (1 serving)

DAY THREE

Breakfast: 2 waffles with strawberries and syrup; 1 cup of skim milk

Snack: Yogurt (1 serving)

Lunch: 1 cup of chili with lean ground beef; 12 ounces of water

Dinner: Fish (preferably baked or grilled); 1 cup of cooked Spanish rice and corn; 12 ounces of water

Snack: Low-fat milkshake

PROGRESS, NOT PERFECTION

We've observed some parents who expect absolute perfection from their kids when it comes to eating. They make their kids egg-white omelets rather than using the whole egg, give them fat-free milk instead of whole milk, and let them snack on fat-free potato chips instead of regular chips. The kids often end up sneaking out for ice cream or bingeing on fried foods at school.

The point we're making is that perfection should be left to those who are perfect. Instead, opt for progress rather than perfection. For instance, if your child loves milk chocolate, give him or her access to it. If you lock it up behind closed pantry doors, your child will simply think of ways to get into the pantry and gorge him or herself. Absolute denial of these comfort foods will often lead to hoarding behaviors in which the child will eat these things secretly. Imagine walking into your child's room and seeing that they've hidden bags of potato chips, candy, and chocolate under the bed. That might happen if you severely restrict your child's eating choices.

You're thinking, "Johnny is getting fat so I better keep these foods away from him." Well, remember, Johnny can still get these foods at school—he can trade his apple for a Twinkie. There's probably a kid in his class that has free access to whatever she wants and doesn't mind eating an apple now and then. For that kid, there's nothing special about Twinkies and other junk foods because her parents give her free access to them.

So, let your child occasionally indulge in junk foods while you emphasize better food choices. Later, your Johnny may start opting for more healthy items to snack on, especially when he realizes that it might affect how he plays sports.

THE FOOD GRADING SCALE

Kids learn early the difference between good and bad, best and second best. One way to instill in a child the value of good eating is to provide him or her with a list of foods that are on the same scale as grades: A = excellent, B = good, C = not-so-good. You'll notice we don't give any foods a failing grade (D or F)—that's because there are no foods or snacks that are inherently bad. We believe that eating one cookie a week is basically harmless, but twenty-five cookies a day might make your kid fat. So, a lot of it depends on the type of food and how much is actually consumed.

So, we'll make it easy for you. Tell your kids to choose foods from the A and B lists at least once or twice per day, assuming that they are eating three regular meals and perhaps having a small snack during the day or at night. Eating A and B foods twice a day is a victory. Remember, don't expect perfection.

How can pretzels be on the C list and avocados on the A list? Pretzels have no fat, and avocados have a lot of fat. But pretzels are a processed food and a high-glycemic carbohydrate (see Chapter 4). For a snack choice, that's bad: pretzels are nutrient-sparse and just not healthy. Avocados, on the other hand, have a lot of healthy fats (unsaturated fats make up more than 80 percent of the fat content), and they contain numerous vitamins and minerals.

In fact, you'll find many high-fat foods on the A list because they contain healthy fats, the mono- and polyunsaturated fats. When we think of all the food choices you can possibly make, eating broiled fish, such as salmon, is the single best choice because it contains quality protein and healthy polyunsaturated fats (EPA and DHA). Also, the wide variety of nuts on the A list, such as peanuts, almonds, and cashews, belong there because of the healthy properties of their fats. So banish forever the notion that eating fat is always bad.

Unfortunately, when you look at the C list, you'll notice that it is filled with the foods that many kids (and adults) eat most. We love our processed foods: the convenience, variety, and taste are great. The problem is, when your diet consists mainly of these foods, you'll end up overweight and sick.

Despite what some nutrition experts have led you to believe, eating boxed cereals is not a healthy choice. Except for cereals containing high-fiber bran, breakfast cereals are mostly sugar. The glycemic index ratings of these cereals are extremely high.

The ABCs of Food

A—Excellent Foods

Almonds
Apples
Avocados
Bananas
Beans (kidney, pinto, and so on)
Berries
Brown rice
Cashews
Chicken and turkey (without the skin)
Corn
Egg whites
Fresh fish (baked, broiled, or grilled; not fried)
Fresh fruits
Grapes
Green vegetables
Macadamia nuts
Mangoes
Oatmeal
Olives
Oranges
Peaches
Peanuts
Pears
Plums
Popcorn (plain)
Raisins
Shellfish
Skim milk
Soy
Tomatoes
Whey and casein
Whole-grain bread

B—Good Foods

Beef, lean cuts
Canned tomato paste
Chocolate*
Frozen veggies and fruits
Grits
Milk (any non-skim milk)
Pork-center tenderloin
Potatoes
Salmon
Sirloin (eye or round and round steak are the leanest cuts)
Spaghetti and sauce
Tuna
Venison
Whole eggs

**Chocolate, especially the dark varieties, has some health benefits due to the presence of antioxidants, which help keep your cells healthy; of course, too much chocolate, because of the high calorie content, may result in body fat gain.*

C—Not-So-Good Foods

Any packaged processed snack
Bacon
Biscuits
Boxed cereal (choose high-fiber, natural cereals; others are mainly sugar)
Bread (white)
Butter
Cake
Chicken and turkey with the skin
Chips
Cookies
Corn dogs
Crackers (saltine)
Fish sticks
Fried chicken
Fried fish
Frozen waffles or pancakes
Hamburgers
Hot dogs
Ice cream
Ketchup
Margarine
Non-dairy creamers
Pancakes
Pastries
Pies
Pizza
Popcorn with butter
Pretzels
Pudding
Sugary juices
Syrup
White rice

And if you add toast with some butter on it, you've got a killer breakfast. High-glycemic, processed white bread slathered with saturated fat from butter is about the worst thing for a child. A better choice would be an omelet (1 whole egg and 2 egg whites with sliced mushrooms, onions, tomatoes, and turkey), a slice of fruit on the side or a small bowl of oatmeal, and a glass of milk (for calcium).

But just because it's on the C list doesn't mean you should eliminate that food completely. Let's face it, everyone loves pizza. The tomato paste on the pizza can actually be quite healthy, even though the processed bread crust isn't the best thing for the body. Your child should be able to eat pizza, though not every day.

SNACKING WISELY

Let your child have his or her favorite junk foods. It's alright for your child occasionally to eat cookies or their favorite piece of pie, muffin, or cake. But at the same time offer him or her a better choice, an A or B choice. For instance, have them snack on nuts of any kind: the fat is healthy and it will satisfy their hunger. Or try slicing up a banana and putting a touch of natural peanut butter on it.

Small fruits like berries (blueberries, strawberries) are great because the volume of food isn't daunting to the child. For instance, some kids might take a bite or two out of an apple, then put it down. Eating the entire apple just isn't going to work for them. But if you leave out blueberries, your child might be more apt to snack on them because they're small, bite-sized pieces. Kids also will imitate your behavior: if they see you eating fresh fruits, nuts, or some other healthy snack, then it will probably leave a permanent impression on them. When your child gets older, he or she will pick up your healthy habits.

Snacks When Traveling

Whenever you take a road trip with your kids, always pack a

snack. In fact, you might find that because their food choices are limited (they're stuck in your car), they may be more apt to eat what you bring. They may beg and plead to stop at the closest fast-food joint, but if you don't pull over, they can't munch on those greasy fries and a burger.

What are good traveling snacks? Nuts of any kind, such as peanuts and cashews, and small bite-size pieces of fruit (such as grapes and berries) are healthy options. Also, you can make sandwiches with whole-grain bread, sliced turkey, mustard, and just a touch of mayonnaise, which will be much healthier than eating fast food. And bring a cooler of bottled water. Eventually, your child will get hungry and the thought of eating grapes will be as wonderful as eating a bag of chocolates.

- *Trail mix*—mixture of cashews, peanuts, raisins, chocolate candies, and so on. The combination of nuts (with healthy fats), raisins (good carbohydrate source), and some fun foods such as chocolates or carob pieces will provide your child with important nutrients, as well as keep him or her from craving other junk foods.

- *Bananas, peaches, plums, pears, carrots*—fruits and vegetables that are easy to carry and convenient to eat. They are excellent snacks for road trips.

- *Peanut butter*—a great source of healthy fats and some protein as well. Peanut butter and jelly sandwiches, though not exactly a healthy food because of the sugar in the jelly, are great for providing calories, healthy fat, and protein to kids.

- *Sports bars*—an excellent and convenient way to get protein and carbohydrates while limiting the consumption of fat.

Snacks at a Game

You've been sitting in the stands watching your eight-year-old play soccer for over an hour. You're tired and hungry and thinking that your kid must be tired and hungry as well. Are there any foods or snacks that might help?

We'd suggest a high-glycemic carbohydrate snack. This could include a sports drink or a carbohydrate-protein bar available at health food stores. Cut up the bars into bite-sized pieces so that it's convenient for your child to eat. Also, stay away from sugar-filled sodas—your child will perform better with a sports drink.

BETTER BAD CHOICES

Let's face it, there will be times when your kid just wants to pig out on pizza dripping in cheese and grease, while drinking a sugar-filled soda. But that's okay: you can't possibly restrict your child's eating around the clock. Here is a concept you might use to convey to your child how food choices should be made—we call it "better bad choices." What this basically means is that when left with choosing two bad foods, pick the one that's less bad. It's still a poor choice, but it's the lesser of two food evils. Below are examples of better bad choices:

BAD CHOICE	BETTER BAD CHOICE
Fried French fries	Baked fries
Fried hamburger on a bun	Grilled hamburger on a bun
Hard candies	Dark chocolate
Hot dog	Low-fat hot dog
Pizza with cheese and cold cuts	Pizza with cheese
Regular greasy potato chips	Baked potato chips
Regular sugar-filled soda	Diet soda
Sugar	Honey

FINAL THOUGHTS

Kids love to snack; in effect, they tend to eat many small meals throughout the day. Interestingly, many athletes do that as well.

So, perhaps, letting your children graze on food all day is better than having them binge during meals.

Remember, let your kids eat from the C list, but try and emphasize the A and B food choices. If you give them the choice, rather than force them, they're more likely to adopt long-term healthy eating habits.

Special Nutritional Needs During Exercise

Your child does not have to be a professional athlete to take advantage of proper pre- and postexercise nutrition, and to do so does not require a nutritionist. Most kids and adolescents have only a fleeting notion of the importance of food, especially when it comes to its impact on exercise and sports. Well, it's about time for that to change. The fundamentals are simple and, once the extraordinary benefits are realized, success will become your child's own motivation to continue.

PRE-EXERCISE NUTRITION

What should your child eat before exercise? We suggest that a meal should be consumed two to three hours before a game or match. Preferably, this meal should contain unprocessed carbohydrates (vegetables and unrefined starches such as oats or brown rice), lean meats (chicken without the skin), and copious amounts of water. It is important as well that your child choose foods that he or she is accustomed to—this is no time to experiment with new food choices. How much your child consumes depends on body weight and age. We do suggest that your child stay away from fatty foods since these take a long time to digest. Plus, your child should consume simple carbohydrates (such as sports drinks) ten minutes or less before the match and keep consuming them throughout the game, when possible.

EATING DURING EXERCISE

Eating during competition is not a bad idea. Usually, the best way to maintain glucose and energy levels is to use sports drinks, so maybe "eating" isn't the right word. During day-long events such as track meets or other activities lasting longer than one hour, consuming 30 grams of carbohydrates per hour may enhance performance. Fruits and crackers (and sports drinks, of course) are ideal choices. Some athletes even consume de-fizzed cola drinks, because the sugar in the cola provides quick energy; however, if your child chooses this route, make sure he or she alternates between de-fizzed cola and water.

POSTEXERCISE REPLENISHMENT

Assuming your kid followed the rules of pre-exercise nutrition, he or she probably just had a career day. So, what do you do? Take your kid home to watch a flick and chill? Not until he or she eats first! Without good nutrition, your child won't recover and the next time out he or she might not be so successful. The first fifteen to thirty minutes following exercise are absolutely crucial. Yes, that's a small window, so come prepared.

If athletes ingest carbohydrates immediately following exercise instead of waiting two hours, they increase glycogen (the stored form of carbohydrates) reserves three to four times faster. This will kick-start the recovery process in your child so he or she is energized for every successive practice, competition, or training session. Specifically, teenage athletes should ingest approximately 0.5 grams of carbohydrates per pound of body weight within fifteen to thirty minutes after exercise. And it goes beyond replenishing energy stores: ingesting fast-acting carbohydrates immediately after exercise can also spur the release of hormones that improve immune function. Also, the carbohydrates given immediately after exercise are instrumental in increasing insulin and growth-hormone levels, which in turn promote muscle growth and recovery (anabolism). A fast-acting carbohydrate is any carbohydrate source abundant in glucose or simple sugars; examples include sports drinks, fruits, breads and bagels, cereals, and fruit bars. Just stay away from high-fat foods and keep the fluids flowing for adequate hydration.

Adding protein to those postexercise carbohydrates will provide the most balanced nutritional replenishment and enhance the insulin and growth-hormone response. Furthermore, glycogen stores are replenished with greater efficiency when protein is added to the mix. Protein should be added to the postexercise meal in a 4:1 ratio of carbohydrates to protein. See the chart below for appropriate amounts of protein and carbohydrates according to body weight.

BODY WEIGHT	CARBOHYDRATES	PROTEIN
88 lbs (40 kg)	40 g	10.0 g
99 lbs (45 kg)	45 g	11.3 g
110 lbs (50 kg)	50 g	12.5 g
121 lbs (55 kg)	55 g	13.8 g
132 lbs (60 kg)	60 g	15.0 g
143 lbs (65 kg)	65 g	16.3 g
154 lbs (70 kg)	70 g	17.5 g
165 lbs (75 kg)	75 g	18.8 g
176 lbs (80 kg)	80 g	20.0 g
187 lbs (85 kg)	85 g	21.3 g
198 lbs (90 kg)	90 g	22.5 g

After a couple of hours, and for the rest of the day, more complex carbohydrates can be ingested with protein. A little fat is allowed as well. Stick to unprocessed carbohydrates, lean proteins, and healthy fats.

Proper postexercise nutrition is really not that difficult, but the difference healthy nutrition can make with young athletes is tremendous. It should *never* be neglected and should be just as much a part of your child's exercise and sporting life as practice,

Common Postexercise Drinks

Many nutrition companies have developed postexercise products for replenishing carbohydrates and protein. Please keep in mind that you should adjust serving size of these products relative to the young athlete's body weight.

PRODUCT	CARB/PROTEIN RATIO	CALORIES
Gatorade Sports Nutrition Shake	4:1	370
Pacific Health Endurox R4	4:1	270
Pacific Health Accelerade	4:1	140

training, and mental preparation. With proper nutrition, peak performance is just a bite away.

THE IMPORTANCE OF HYDRATION

As a parent of an athletic child, the last thing you want to see is your kid sprawled out on the playing field, writhing in pain from injury. It's never comforting, but just think how much worse it could be without pads, proper technique, and good coaching; although they cannot guarantee injury prevention, they certainly make a substantial difference. But what about protection against other stressors? What are the pads for the internal organs and delicate molecular functions that are central to all the body's functions? Specifically, what will guard against heat stress? While injuries are scary, there is nothing more frightening than "total system failure."

Heat-related injuries have unfortunately found their way into the headlines in recent years as a handful of heat-related deaths have rocked the athletic world. Heat stroke is the second leading cause of death in high-school athletes.[1] Even in professional

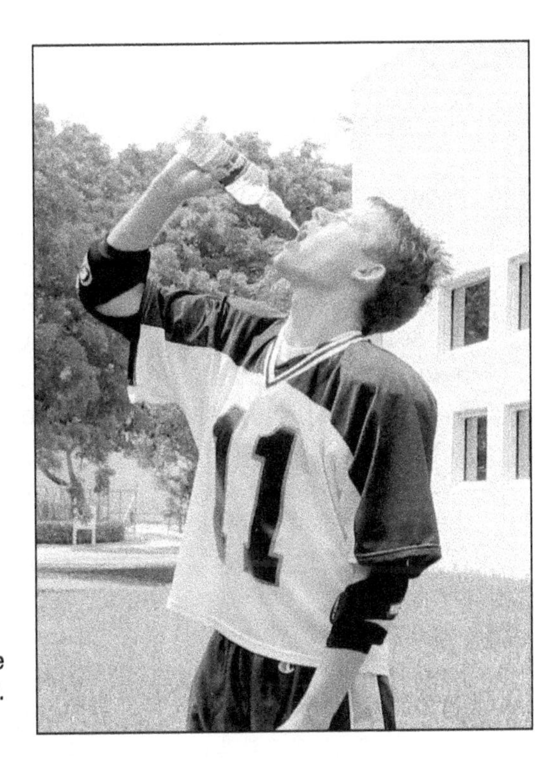

Staying hydrated while exercising is critical.

sports, under the watch of the most well-trained doctors and training staffs, athletes routinely fall ill to heat exhaustion. In kids, the risks are even greater.

Children tolerate temperature extremes less efficiently than adults and have a lower sweating rate, making it even more difficult to rid excess heat from the body. When they exercise, the heat transfer from the muscles to the skin is poor, making kids more prone to overheating.

Even before dehydration occurs a decline in performance is likely. Just a 2 percent reduction in body weight from fluid loss can lead to a significant decline in muscular strength and endurance.[2] That's a mere 2 pounds for a 100-pound athlete, after which you may expect dizziness, headaches, and extreme fatigue.

Preventing Dehydration

An extremely important detail to remember is that thirst is not a

Invasion of the Sports Drink

Besides water, what types of fluids should be ingested and are they any better than water? Well, water certainly works well, but to promote the willingness to drink, beverages should be tasty and stimulate thirst. Sports drinks can help because kids seem to prefer fruit-flavored drinks. Studies have demonstrated that sports drinks keep children better hydrated than drinking plain or flavored water. The additional carbohydrates in sports drinks reduce dehydration to a greater extent than water, and the extra sodium helps the small intestine "suck in" more fluids.[3]

Specifically, sports drinks should be 6 to 8 percent carbohydrate. This amount is not only readily absorbed into the bloodstream, but when imbibed in proper amounts, the added carbohydrates aid in performance and endurance. Drinks consisting of less than 5 percent carbohydrate do not provide enough energy to improve performance; drinks with higher percentages, like some that are 10 to 12 percent carbohydrate, open the possibility of stomach upset and impaired performance. The 6 to 8 percent level amounts to about 15–18 grams of carbohydrate per cup of sports drink.

As far as the type of carbohydrate, glucose, glucose polymers (maltodextrin), and sucrose all fare equally well. Just stay away from high amounts of fructose, as it can cause diarrhea. Also, avoid undiluted juice or carbonated sodas since these contain too much carbohydrate and may cause stomach upset.

Caffeine should also be avoided because it actually promotes fluid loss through urination. In children, it can also be associated with agitation, nausea, and headaches.[4] Obviously, none of these side effects will help their performance. Even after activity, caffeine is not recommended because it may inhibit the rehydration process.

Small amounts of sodium, on the other hand, can be advantageous for fluid absorption. Sodium is usually contained in sports drinks. You can also give your kid saltine crackers. The salt will make him or her want to drink more, resulting in the intake of both salt and fluid. Salt tablets, however, should be avoided entirely, as they can cause nausea and irritation of the stomach lining. Also, they actually contribute to dehydration by causing water to be pulled away from body tissues that need it. This explains the muscle cramps that often occur with the use of salt tablets.

POPULAR FLUID-REPLACEMENT BEVERAGES

BEVERAGE (8 OZ)	CARBOHYDRATE	PERCENT CONCENTRATION	SODIUM/ POTASSIUM
Accelerade	sucrose/ maltodextrin	7.7	190 mg/64 mg
AllSport	fructose	8.0	55 mg/55 mg
Coca-Cola	fructose/sucrose	11.0	6 mg/trace
Gatorade	sucrose/glucose	6.0	110 mg/30 mg
Orange juice	fructose/sucrose	10.0	64 mg/36 mg
Powerade	fructose/ maltodextrin	8.0	55 mg/30 mg
Water	none	none	low/low

good indicator of a child's need for fluids. If they're thirsty during athletic competition or training, they've already entered the first stage of dehydration. From there, the situation can become quite dire. So, special emphasis should be placed on ensuring adequate fluid intake before, during, and after physical activity. Many children and adults do not drink enough fluids during activity, but a child's core temperature will rise faster than an adult's, and kids don't often recognize the symptoms of heat strain. Given their

Recognizing and Treating Heat Disorders

Heat illness—*Signs and symptoms:* weakness, chills, nausea, headache, faintness, disorientation, muscle cramping/pain/spasms, fatigue, bright or dark urine or small volume of urine. *Response/treatment:* move child to the shade, remove excess clothing, have child drink 4–8 ounces of fluid (preferably a sports drink) every ten to fifteen minutes; add salt to foods.

Heat exhaustion—*Signs and symptoms:* nausea, extreme fatigue, reduced sweating, headache, shortness of breath, weak and rapid pulse, dry mouth. *Response/treatment:* move child to a cool place, have child drink 16 ounces of fluid (preferably a sports drink) for every pound of weight lost, remove sweaty clothes, place ice behind the head; may require medical attention.

Heat stroke—*Signs and symptoms:* lack of sweating, dry and hot skin, swollen tongue, visual disturbances, rapid pulse, loss of balance, fainting, vomiting, loss of consciousness, shock. *Response/treatment:* requires immediate medical attention—call 911; remove sweaty clothes, cover child in ice packs, immerse in cold water, elevate feet.[5]

competitive nature, some kids may inadvertently push themselves into a heat-related illness.

Of course, weather that is hot and dry can be extremely dangerous. Because sweat evaporates very quickly in such conditions, your child may not feel sweaty and you probably will not recognize how much water he or she has lost. Also dangerous is high humidity: sweat drips off the skin so that the cooling benefit of evaporation is lost even at lower temperatures, resulting in a buildup of body heat that can lead to heat stress.

Even in water and winter sports, proper hydration is a must. A swimmer still loses body fluids through sweat in the pool and can become dehydrated just by sitting and waiting to compete in the hot, humid environment of a swim meet. Winter sports athletes (figure skaters, hockey players, skiers) also may not realize the importance of fluid replacement because they practice and play in a cool or cold environment. Actually, because clothing and equipment reduces the ability of the body to cool itself, heat stress is also likely in winter sports, making proper hydration even more crucial.

Preventing dehydration is simple: A good start is to provide children with a personalized water bottle and encouraging them to drink at regular intervals. A common suggestion is to have a child drink until he or she is not thirsty, and then drink an additional half-glass of liquid. More specifically, children should plan on drinking 8 ounces of water, fruit juice, or sports drink an hour or two before physical activity begins. Then, about ten to twenty minutes before the activity, an additional 4 ounces should be ingested. You can double these totals for adolescents.

During exercise, children should drink 3–4 ounces of water, diluted juice, or sports drink every fifteen minutes; for adolescents, that amount increases to 4–8 ounces every fifteen minutes. But even that may not be enough. Since children do not instinctively drink enough fluids to replace water losses, their intake needs to be monitored. Therefore, it's essential that you watch how much water they actually drink. Finally, after exercise, both children and adolescents should ingest 2 cups of water for every pound of weight lost. Also, a copious intake of carbohydrate-containing liquids is recommended to promote recovery.

Guidelines for Fluid Replacement

Children (5–11 years old)

Before exercise: Drink 8 ounces of water, fruit juice, or sports drink, one to two hours before activity. Also, drink 4–8 ounces of water, fruit juice, or sports drink, ten to twenty minutes before activity.

During exercise: Drink 3–4 ounces of water every fifteen minutes. After one hour of continuous exercise, drink diluted juice, sports drink, or water.

After exercise: Drink 2 cups of water for every pound of weight loss from exercise; liberal intake of carbohydrate-containing fluids.

Adolescents (11–18 years old)

Before exercise: Drink 8–16 ounces of water, fruit juice, or sports drink, one to two hours before activity. Also, drink 8–12 ounces of water, fruit juice, or sports drink, ten to twenty minutes before activity.

During exercise: Drink 4–8 ounces of water every fifteen minutes. After one hour of continuous exercise, drink diluted juice, sports drink, or water.

After exercise: Drink 2 cups of water for every pound of weight lost through exercise; liberal intake of carbohydrate-containing fluids.[6]

Preventing Heat Disorders

Avoiding dehydration in children goes beyond ingesting enough fluids. Children also adjust poorly to hot environments and therefore need to increase their level of exercise intensity slowly (over a period of five to ten days). This makes the duty of coaches and parents all the more important, but much of it is simple common sense:

- Schedule frequent rest periods and water breaks in the shade.
- Cancel or reschedule practice to avoid the hottest times of the day.

- Modify drills and clothing to prevent overheating.
- Weigh athletes before and after practice to estimate their water loss.
- Be aware of those kids that are obese, poorly conditioned, or have health problems. These kids are at an increased risk of heat disorders, as are athletes who are trying to lose weight, such as wrestlers, gymnasts, and dancers. They often engage in dangerous dehydration techniques that should never be encouraged.
- Finally, *never* restrict fluids.

Luckily, heat stress is readily preventable if these guidelines are followed. It is unfortunate, and sometimes deadly, when they are not. A child's health should always be the primary focus when engaging in athletic activities. Maintaining proper hydration should be as obvious and practical as it is to wear a helmet when playing football. By following these simple rules, the focus can shift back to what really counts—having fun.

Tips for Gaining and Losing Weight

Kids these days are getting hit from all angles—if not physically on the football field or basketball court, they're bombarded by peer pressure and media messages of who and what they should be. At earlier ages than ever before, they become concerned with—even obsessed by—their physical appearance. It seems, for young girls, that the emphasis on being thin is reaching epidemic proportions. According to the National Eating Disorders Association, an estimated 51 percent of girls ages nine to ten feel better about themselves if they are on a diet. For young boys, the pressure to gain muscle and dominate opposing athletes is now evident on every level of play. What often gets lost in the desire to lose or gain weight is how to do it the right way—the healthy way.

No ten-year-old is going to have the emotional maturity to develop and maintain a proper diet and exercise regimen. Children may only know that "thin is in" or be concerned with how much they can bench press. There is a *right* way to gain weight and a *right* way to lose weight, and ultimately it's up to the parents to instill healthy habits.

GAINING WEIGHT THE HEALTHY WAY

It's a fact that gaining weight can give young athletes the competitive edge to excel in their chosen sport. A child who is too thin to compete can benefit from a dietary regimen and exercise program that promotes gains in lean body mass. To gain weight, children simply need to consume more calories than what is normally expended for activity and growth. Those extra calories will add body weight, but to ensure that it doesn't turn to fat, exercise is mandatory. However, and this is extremely important, children do not have the hormones to rapidly build larger and stronger muscles *until they reach puberty.* Too many parents mistakenly assume that their child is exercising or eating improperly if he's not busting out of his shirts every six months. Give it time: some kids need to grow into their frames, and they won't do it significantly until puberty.

Above all else, be realistic. A registered dietician or physician can recommend a body weight goal and from there your child can slowly work on reaching it. The progress should be gradual to ensure less body-fat gains. Specifically, no more than half a pound should be gained each week. Since it takes 2,500 calories to add a pound of muscle, you only need 1,250 extra calories per week to

Fit Kids Strategies for Gaining Weight

- Encourage your child to increase portion sizes and snack regularly throughout the day.
- Stay away from fatty foods and fried foods.
- Use resistance training to add muscle.
- Eat a large meal toward the end of the day.
- Eat healthy foods that consist mainly of unprocessed carbohydrates, healthy fats, and lean proteins.
- Use supplements such as protein shakes, if needed (liquid meals are very convenient).

reach this goal. Divided over seven days, that's only 179 extra calories per day—basically, the equivalent of a small sandwich.

Of course, a child may still burn off this extra amount since, typically, children are so incredibly active. That's why you need to have your child step on that scale every week, at the same time, wearing the same amount of clothes, to monitor and modify progress. Not seeing any gains? Then you and your kid need to spend more time in the kitchen.

Generally, the extra calories should come from healthy foods such as unprocessed carbohydrates (oatmeal, whole-grain breads, vegetables, fruits), unsaturated fats (peanuts or unprocessed peanut butter, nuts such as cashews and almonds), and lean proteins (chicken without the skin, baked fish, lean cuts of beef and pork). We know the RDA of 0.8 grams of protein is inadequate for exercising adults; thus it would be sensible to have a child eat at least 0.6–0.9 grams of protein per pound of body weight. Although the number of required calories varies considerably from child to child, in general children who exercise and compete at high levels need to eat as much as 3,000–4,000 calories daily.

Clearly, if the child's basic energy needs are not being met through his or her normal diet, then eating any and all foods may be warranted (though this won't necessarily foster good eating habits). If that's the case, make sure your child takes a children's multivitamin to ensure that he or she meets the minimal daily requirements for micronutrients.

LOSING WEIGHT THE HEALTHY WAY

A child who is overweight, or even one who has the false perception of being overweight, can have a damaged outlook on life and food that persists for life. Children need energy to perform and function properly, and food is the only thing that provides it. Severely restricting food intake can be disastrous to the health of a child. So, just as with gaining weight, losing it should be a slow, gradual process. Likewise, some kids just need to grow taller or reach puberty before their bodies take on their intended form.

If you think your child is overweight, consult with your physician or a registered dietician. They can prescribe a realistic weight goal for your child's age and developmental level. And before we get into specifics for losing weight, remember to be a role model yourself: eat a healthy, well-balanced diet, take an active role in the pursuit of fitness and health, and exercise! That alone will do wonders for your child's outlook on food, fitness, and body image.

Remember that losing weight is not a matter of being "on a diet"; it's a lifestyle change. So, on a permanent basis, replace high-sugar, high-fat foods with nutrient-dense, unprocessed foods. This will improve your child's energy stores so he or she can burn off excess fat through exercise. Aerobic exercises—such as run-

Fit Kids Strategies for Losing Weight

- In general, approximately half a pound of weight should be lost per week.
- Work with a registered dietician to determine caloric requirements for your child. A dietician will take into account age, gender, weight, and the intensity, frequency, and duration of physical activity—all of which will dictate the young athlete's energy needs.
- The initial weight-loss goal should not exceed 10 percent of body weight.
- Your child should do an aerobic activity, such as fast walking, running, biking, and swimming, two to three times per week for thirty minutes.
- Food should be eaten at regular intervals—three meals daily, plus two nutrient-dense snacks.
- Your child should drink at least 8 ounces of water before every meal.

ning, biking, and swimming—are excellent for losing fat and burning calories.

Just don't get hung up on your child losing a specific amount of weight over a certain amount of time, because this may set him or her up for failure. Remember, weight loss should be gradual—no more than half a pound a week. Promoting a healthy lifestyle is more important than how fast a child drops the pounds.

Promoting a healthy lifestyle is more important than how fast a child drops the pounds.

As for specific foods, focus on low-fat milk products, lean meats and fish, fruits, vegetables, and plenty of whole-grain breads, and pasta. Keep the gravy, butter, and sauces to a minimum (that goes for parents, too!). Also, cut back on foods with empty calories, such as candy bars, chips, cookies, and sodas. Replace them with fruits, bran cereals, granola bars, and pastas. Eat as a family and don't single out a child by restricting foods or telling the child he or she is on a special diet; portion control is the key. And eat at regular intervals: don't be afraid to have your child eat five smaller meals per day, as this is beneficial for increasing metabolism and avoiding wild, impulsive bouts of eating.

Changing behaviors is also critical: get your child away from the TV while eating, because he or she will eat more in front of the tube. According to a study in *Pediatrics,* increased television viewing is associated with being overweight.[1] That means the more your child sits in front of the TV, the less he or she will be doing something active and the greater the chance of becoming overweight. Finally, get your kid to take the stairs, do more chores around the house, walk to school if it's realistic, and play with the neighborhood kids every day.

The Pitfalls of Weight Loss

As a parent, you may stress the importance of weight loss to your child as a means to improved health and long-term well-being, but your child may not see it that way. Most children do not look beyond a month or so into the future, and most feel they are healthy regardless of their body type. They are, however, motivated by concerns about self-esteem and appearance. And it begins early: almost half of girls in the first and second grades want to be thinner.[2] And an estimated 40 to 60 percent of high-school girls are on diets.[3] Young women, especially, tend to view thinness as more important than fitness. And if they feel healthy, they assume that they are healthy. This combination may lead to the development of an eating disorder, such as anorexia nervosa or bulimia.

Perhaps the most difficult task facing parents whose child may have an eating disorder is breaking down their child's self-imposed barriers about his or her appearance. One of the hallmarks of an eating disorder is secrecy and denial, which makes identification and treatment a challenge. The psychology behind an eating disorder is extremely complicated and not well understood. Regardless of what you may tell your child about his or her appearance, he or she still feels overweight and unattractive. Unfortunately, eating disorders are now seen at earlier ages than ever before. The best defense, of course, is preventing disorders from ever taking root.

How do you do that? Regardless of whether an eating disorder appears imminent or not, caloric intake should not fall lower than 2,000 calories per day when striving for weight loss. Through appropriate exercise, a negative daily caloric deficit (more calories expended than ingested) is possible. Weight loss should be extended and slow, and no weight cycling (repeated weight loss and regain) should occur. Weight cycling can be detrimental to metabolism, performance, and health. After all, it's easy to drop a few pounds in a day if you just don't eat. The loss is all water weight, but impressionable adolescents may love seeing the pounds come off the scale, and this only reinforces negative behavior. Pretty soon, they're in a cycle that's extremely difficult to break and, just like that, an eating disorder is established.

It's important to realize that seemingly innocent, even playful, comments about weight can be interpreted incorrectly by children and adolescents. Kids are eager to please and they especially want to please their parents and friends. Being ridiculed or singled out for having a weight problem can be devastating: just one instance can trigger unhealthy eating habits and lead to a disorder. In addition, using food as a reward or punishment should be avoided. Try not to say things like "you better finish what's on your plate before I let you go out and play." Let your child eat until he or she is satisfied, and don't force your child to eat. This just creates emotional issues about eating and food.

Excessive and rapid weight loss is the most telling sign of an eating disorder. Other signs include preoccupation with food and exercise, denial of hunger, frequent weighing, evidence of binge eating and self-induced vomiting, use of drugs such as laxatives and diuretics, and mood swings.

Treatment of eating disorders is difficult, but it has become a specialty involving a team of professionals, including doctors, dieticians, psychologists, trainers, and coaches. Of course, parents play as big a role as anyone. After a private intervention and the child's recognition and confession of a problem, treatment can begin by setting realistic goals for body composition and weight. Love, and a supportive environment, should not be in short supply. For more information on eating disorders and what to look for and do, contact the National Eating Disorders Association (see Resources).

Conclusion

Young athletes and fitness enthusiasts should have one thing clear from the start: Exercise and eating right are the best ways to promote health and well-being. Impressionable young children need guidance and support, and the best place to get it is from parents and coaches. Promoting and encouraging physical perfection, or rewarding it excessively, can send a message that is inappropriate and occasionally tragic. Seek perfection as a team in practice, in eating for health, and in promoting fun. Fun and lifelong health are the true rewards.

Parents can play a significant role in keeping their children fit and healthy. Good nutrition and exercise learned as a child can mean a long and active life as an adult. We hope that this book will help you foster these healthy habits in your children, and to further that end we'd like to review some of the basic concepts we've presented in the form of questions and answers.

Q: Is lifting weights safe for a young child?

A: Yes, weight lifting is safe. What comes as a surprise to most parents is that activities like running and jumping—things your child probably performs on a daily basis—are likely to stress the body to a greater extent than weight training and result in more frequent injuries. This book provides overall guidance for weight training, but you should also consult a personal trainer or a strength and conditioning professional, who can teach your child the proper techniques of weight training. For those just beginning weight lifting, technique is of primary importance. If a child never learns the proper lifting techniques, then he or she is more susceptible to injury.

At what age can a child start lifting weights? The simple answer is—at any age he or she wants, as long as adult supervision is present.

Q: What are some of the benefits of exercise for kids?

A: Exercise and sports offer social relationships, physical challenges, and honest competition. There is evidence that playing sports can increase a child's self-esteem and academic performance, while decreasing the likelihood of disease. For example, many of the risk factors for cardiovascular disease are already present in childhood and early adolescence. Fortunately, regular physical exercise can help to diminish, or nearly eliminate, these risk factors. Additionally, weight training can provide stronger bones, enhanced strength, and improved athletic ability.

The social and psychological benefits of sports participation are almost too numerous to count. How can you possibly measure the value and satisfaction derived from working hard and mastering a skill? Participating in sports also allows children to take on leadership roles, handle adversity, and improve their time management—qualities important for succeeding in adulthood.

Q: What exactly is an appropriate weight-training regimen for young athletes?

A: It is important to be aware that the most common injuries among children who weight train are joint strains and muscle strains of the low back. While this is usually caused by poor technique, a lack of "core" training may also be the culprit. Core training, which involves general strengthening of the muscles surrounding the abdomen and low back, should be a top priority for young athletes who lift weights. The core is the "hub" or base of operations for the extremities; without a strong core, an athlete is more likely to suffer muscle imbalances and injury. Also, because the core muscles transfer power from the legs to the upper body, and vice versa, developing the core is extremely important for playing sports.

When a child is mentally and physically prepared to start weight training, exercises should focus on proper technique—keeping weight moderate and using a high number of repetitions (10–20). Balance should be promoted, maximal loads must be avoided, and stretching and calisthenics need to be incorporated.

Q: My child is already active in sports, but how do I make sure she is getting all the right foods to keep her active?

A: Physical activity takes its toll: the more kids exercise and participate in sports, the more calories and nutrients they need. They already need a lot of calories for proper growth, but sports activities place tremendous additional demands on the respiratory, cardiovascular, muscular, and skeletal systems.

Do not restrict foods based on their fat content. Fat is a major source of energy, especially in children and adolescents, and provides most of the fuel for endurance events. Fat is also essential for hormone production, and sources of fat usually contain increased levels of important nutrients such as iron, protein, and calcium. Stay away from junk foods and foods high in saturated fats (these should make up no more than 10 percent of total calories). Also, encourage kids to drink plenty of fluids before, during, and after exercise, and have them consume additional carbohydrates about one hour before exercise or sporting events lasting longer than ninety minutes. As always, encourage kids to eat breakfast and promote healthy snacking; this ensures adequate energy that will last throughout the day.

Maintaining a proper diet today will not only provide energy for your child's current sports participation, but it will also have a striking impact on her health throughout adolescence and adulthood. She is more likely to continue healthy eating habits and thereby prevent disease processes.

Q: What about "junk food" for kids? Should they have free access to junk food, have it on a limited basis, or should I completely eliminate these foods from the household?

A: First of all, even if you eradicate all junk food from your house, kids will still see those foods at their school, at their friends' homes, at the mall, and at movie theaters. Your child may end up bingeing on the stuff when he or she is outside your home. Eliminate the allure of these good-for-the-taste-buds but bad-for-the-body treats by letting your child have junk foods, but try to emphasize the value of good foods as well. Eventually, your kids will be adept enough at purchasing their own foods—go to any mall and see kids eating pizza, burgers, and sodas. Hopefully, you can instill in them the value of good eating. Then, even if they pig out on junk food one day, the next day they'll eat a healthy salad, fruit, and some lean cuts of protein-filled meat.

Q: Should teenagers be taking dietary supplements?

A: The fact is that most of us do not eat perfectly. Having your teenager take a multivitamin won't replace proper eating habits, but at least he or she will get the nutrients that may otherwise be missing in the diet. After all, most supplements are derived from food and, thus, they are just as healthy as (if not more healthy than) what is served on your dinner table. However, supplementation should always be a second choice—eating the right foods is clearly the number-one goal.

What about other supplements such as protein powders, energy bars, or protein shakes? Again, it's best to encourage your child to get protein from unprocessed foods such as chicken, turkey, lean cuts of beef, and fish. But if given the choice between an unhealthy snack laden with fat and sugar or a protein shake, go with the shake. Supplements for gaining weight or protein supplements are terrific additions if the teen is already eating a healthy diet. Just make sure your young athlete is exercising or involved in rigorous sporting activity. Also, stay away from the "hormone-related" supplements (such as andro and norandro).

Q: What should my kid eat while she's playing sports? She's out there for hours—is there anything she might have to help her maintain energy levels?

A: First of all, make sure your child is hydrated. It is extremely important to remember that thirst is not a good indicator of a child's need for fluids. If a child is thirsty during athletic competition or training, he or she has already entered the first stage of dehydration. Have her drink water or a sports beverage before and during the game. During exercise, children should drink 3–4 ounces of water, diluted juice, or sports drink every fifteen minutes; for adolescents, that amount increases to 4–8 ounces.

There are a number of good sports nutrition bars (containing mainly carbohydrates, protein, and fat) that she can snack on when she's resting. For instance, cut up a nutrition bar into bite-sized pieces and have her consume one when she's on the sideline. During day-long events such as track meets or other activities lasting longer than one hour, consuming 30 grams of carbohydrates per hour may enhance performance. Fruits and crackers (and sports drinks, of course) are ideal choices. Some athletes even consume de-fizzed cola drinks, because the sugar in the cola provides quick energy; however, if your child chooses this method, she should alternate between de-fizzed cola and water.

Q: What about "carbohydrate loading" for marathon runners? Since fats carry 9 calories per gram and carbohydrates have only 4 calories, why not load up with fats instead?

A: Carbohydrates remain the ideal choice for energy because they can be utilized more efficiently by the body than fats. Fats provide twice the energy of carbs, but to be oxidized (burned for energy) they need about 75 percent more oxygen during strenuous activity. As you know, taking in a lot of extra oxygen is very difficult when you're running a marathon. Carbohydrates, on the other hand, are readily converted to glycogen and used for energy.

Q: Is postexercise nutrition important? What types of foods should children eat?

A: Proper postexercise dietary intake is critical and has become one of the most actively researched areas of sports nutrition. Put simply, your body is craving nutrients after a workout, and it will utilize them most effectively during this period. There is roughly a two-hour window after exercise when the body will most efficiently replenish itself—enough time for a protein/carbohydrate drink immediately after training and a healthy meal not long after that.

Young athletes should ingest carbohydrates and protein in a 3:1 ratio immediately after training or competition. With endurance exercises, the ratio can be higher; if mainly doing weight-training exercises, the ratio should be lower. Consume carbohydrates at 1 gram per kilogram of body weight (0.45 grams per pound). So, for a 100-pound athlete, that amounts to 45 grams of carbohydrates. Using the 3:1 ratio, you will also need to add 15 grams of protein. Keep fat-intake low, so as not to interfere with digestion. Also, for faster digestion and utilization, liquid meals work best and whey protein is ideal. Fast-acting carbohydrates (simple sugars, grape juice, and yogurt with fruit) are optimal.

The next meal should be similar, with even more calories overall. Fat content can be a little higher and lean sources of protein will promote muscle recovery. Also, eat slow-acting carbohydrates, such as potatoes, pastas, and breads.

Q: Is it safe to put a young child on a diet?

A: Unfortunately, obesity is becoming more prevalent in this country. If you think your child is overweight, consult with your physician or a registered dietician. They can prescribe a realistic weight goal for your child's age and developmental level. However, restricting a child's food choices at a young age will likely lead to food cravings, the hoarding of food, and may start a never-ending cycle of perpetual dieting. Instead, lead by example: let the child see how and what you eat, and let them watch how you exercise. Children repeat almost everything they see their parents do. If your child sees that you can take a bite or two of cake and not go hog-wild eating half the cake, then again your child will follow your example. And let's face it, if your idea of strenuous exercise is wrestling with the cookie jar, then your child will probably have the same mindset.

Another important reason not to put children on a diet is because they are growing. They need calories—protein, fat, and carbohydrates—in order to feed their growing bones, muscles, and organs. Have your child eat whole eggs, drink skim milk, and encourage him or her to eat vegetables. If your child sees you eat healthy foods, perhaps he or she will pick up the same healthy habit.

Remember that losing weight is not a matter of being "on a diet"; it's a lifestyle change. So, on a permanent basis, replace high-sugar, high-fat foods with nutrient-dense, unprocessed foods. This will improve your child's energy stores so he or she can burn off excess fat through exercise. Aerobic exercises—such as running, biking, and swimming—are excellent for helping kids lose fat and burn calories.

Resources

INFORMATION ON FITNESS AND EXERCISE FOR CHILDREN AND BEGINNERS

Books

Strength and Power for Young Athletes by A. Faigenbaum and W. Westcott (Champaign, IL: Human Kinetics, 2000).

Strength Training for Young Athletes by W. Kraemer and S. Fleck (Champaign, IL: Human Kinetics, 1993).

Other Resources

The Governor's Council on Physical Fitness, Health, and Sports and The Michigan Fitness Foundation
P.O. Box 27187
Lansing, MI 48909
Tel: 517-347-7891 or 800-434-8642
Website: www.michiganfitness.org

MomsTeam: Youth Sports Information for Parents
MomsTeam Media
60 Thoreau Street, Suite 288
Concord, MA 01742
Website: www.MomsTeam.com

National Alliance for Youth Sports
2050 Vista Parkway
West Palm Beach, FL 33411
Tel: 561-684-1141 or 800-688-KIDS
Website: www.nays.org

The President's Council on Physical Fitness and Sports
Department W
200 Independence Avenue, SW, Room 738-H
Washington, D.C. 20201-0004
Tel: 202-690-9000
Website: www.fitness.gov

SportingKid: The Magazine for Families with Active Lifestyles
240 Prospect Place, Unit E1
Alpharetta, GA 30005
Tel: 678-297-3903
Website: www.sportingkid.com

Youth Sport Trust
Sir John Beckwith Centre for Sport
Loughborough University
Loughborough
Leicestershire LE11 3TU
Website: www.youthsporttrust.org

INFORMATION ON NUTRITION FOR YOUNG ATHLETES

Books

Child Health, Nutrition, and Physical Activity by L. Cheung and J. Richmond (Champaign, IL: Human Kinetics, 1995).

Fuel for Young Athletes by A. Litt (Champaign, IL: Human Kinetics, 2003).

Play Hard Eat Right by D. Jennings and S. Steen (Minneapolis, MN: Chronimed Publishing, 1995).

Other Resources

National Eating Disorders Association
603 Stewart Street, Suite 803
Seattle, WA 98101
Tel: 206-382-3587
Website: www.nationaleatingdisorders.org

International Society of Sports Nutrition (ISSN)
600 Pembrook Drive
Woodland Park, CO 80863
Tel: 866-472-4650
Website: www.sportsnutritionsociety.org

HOW TO FIND A QUALIFIED TRAINER

American Council on Exercise (ACE)
4851 Paramount Drive
San Diego, CA 92123
Tel: 858-279-8227 or 800-825-3636
Website: www.acefitness.org/profreg/default.aspx

IDEAfit.com
Website: www.ideafit.com/trainerlocator.asp

National Strength and Conditioning Association
P.O. Box 9908
Colorado Springs, CO 80932
Tel: 719-632-6722 or 800-815-6826
E-mail: nsca@nsca-lift.org
Website: www.nsca-lift.org

Notes

Introduction: Fit Kids Become Fit Adults

1. P.H. Walters et al., "Childhood Obesity: Causes and Treatment," *Health & Fitness Journal* 7:1 (2003): 1722.

2. Ibid.

3. Results of an A.C. Nielsen survey, published by Reuters, August 11, 2003.

Chapter 1: The Benefits of Exercise and Sports Participation for Kids

1. T. Dwyer, F. Sallis, L. Blizzard et al., "Relation of Academic Performance to Physical Activity and Fitness in Children," *Pediatric Exercise Science* 13 (2001): 225–237; R.J. Gretebeck, R.E. Kappes, and P.H. Kulinna, "Sports Participation and Lifestyle Behaviors in Adolescents," ACSM National Conference (2002).

2. M.S. Sothern, M. Loftin, R.M. Suskind et al., "The Health Benefits of Physical Activity in Children and Adolescents: Implications for Chronic Disease Prevention," *European Journal of Pediatrics* 158:4 (1999): 271–274.

3. T. Housh, D. Housh, and H. DeVries, *Applied Exercise and Sport Physiology* (Scottsdale, AZ: Holcomb Hathaway, 2002).

4. T. Dwyer, F. Sallis, L. Blizzard et al., "Relation of Academic Performance" (see n. 1); R.J. Gretebeck, R.E. Kappes, and P.H. Kulinna, "Sports Participation and Lifestyle Behaviors" (see n. 1).

5. National Strength and Conditioning Association, "Youth Resistance Training" (see n. 2).

6. Women's Sports Foundation, 305-315 Hither Green Lane, Lewisham, London SE13 6TJ; website: www.wsf.org.uk.

7. National Strength and Conditioning Association, "Youth Resistance Training" (see n. 2).

8. H. Kemper, "Skeletal Development during Childhood and Adolescence" (see n. 2); National Strength and Conditioning Association, "Youth Resistance Training" (see n. 2).

9. Ibid.

10. H. Kemper, "Skeletal Development during Childhood and Adolescence" (see n. 2).

11. L. Wiersma, "Risks and Benefits of Youth Sport Specialization: Perspectives and Recommendations," *Pediatric Exercise Science* 12 (2000): 13–22.

12. Ibid.

13. Faigenbaum, AD, Westcott, WL, Loud, RL, and Long C. The Effect of different resistance training protocols of musclular strength and endurance development in children. *Pediatrics* (1999) 104:e5-e9.]

14. National Strength and Conditioning Association, "Youth Resistance Training" (see n. 2).

15. Ibid.

Chapter 2: Simple Rules of Exercise for Kids

1. National Strength and Conditioning Association, "Youth Resistance Training" (see ch. 1, n. 2).

2. Ibid.

3. R.C. Stucky-Ropp and T.M. DiLorenzo, "Determinants of Exercise in Children," *Preventive Medicine* 22:6 (1993): 880–889.

4. L. Moore et al., "Influence of Parents' Physical Activity Levels on Activity Levels of Young Children," *Journal of Pediatrics* 118 (1991): 215–219.

5. R. Klesges et al., "Effects of Obesity, Social Interactions, and Physical Environment on Physical Activity in Preschoolers," *Health Psychology* 9 (1990): 435–449.

6. M. Fogelholm et al., "Parent-Child Relationship of Physical Activity

Patterns and Obesity," *International Journal of Obesity* 23 (1999): 1262–1268.

Chapter 3: Strength Training and Conditioning for Children

1. D. Baker, "Science and Practice of Coaching a Strength Training Program for Novice and Intermediate-level Athletes," *Strength and Conditioning* 23:2 (2001): 61–68.

2. S.J. Fleck and W.J. Kraemer, "Children and Resistance Training," in *Designing Resistance Training Programs* 2nd ed., 199–216 (Champaign, IL: Human Kinetics, 1987).

Chapter 4: Basic Nutrition for Fit Kids

1. *Teens & Sports Participation in America 2001* (North Palm Beach, FL: SGMA, 2001).

2. J.M. Foricher et al., "Effects of Submaximal Intensity Cycle Ergometery for One Hour on Substrate Utilization in Trained Pubertal Boys versus Trained Adults," *Journal of Sports Medicine and Physical Fitness* 43 (2003): 36–43.

3. J.L. Thompson, "Energy Balance in Young Athletes," *International Journal of Sports Nutrition* 8 (1998): 160–174.

4. V. Matkovic, "Calcium and Peak Bone Mass," *Journal of Internal Medicine* 23:2 (1992): 151–160.

5. S.J. Stear, A. Prentice, S.C. Jones, and T.J. Cole, "Effect of Calcium and Exercise Intervention on the Bone Mineral Status of 16- to 18-year-old Adolescent Girls," *American Journal of Clinical Nutrition* 77 (2003): 985–992.

6. P.D. Delmas, "Treatment of Postmenopausal Osteoporosis," *The Lancet* 359:9322 (2002): 2018–2026.

7. J.L. Thompson, "Energy Balance in Young Athletes," *International Journal of Sports Nutrition* 8 (1998): 160–174.

8. P. Ziegler, R. Sharp, V. Hughes et al., "Nutritional Status of Teenage Female Competitive Figure Skaters," *Journal of the American Dietetic Association* 102 (2002): 374–379.

9. B. Friedman, E. Weller, H. Mairbaurl, and P. Bartsch, "Effects of Iron

Repletion on Blood Volume and Performance Capacity in Young Athletes," *Medicine and Science in Sports and Exercise* 33 (2001): 741–746.

10. S.M. Kleiner, *Power Eating* (Champaign, IL: Human Kinetics, 2001), 141.

11. Bar-Or Oded, "Nutritional Considerations for the Child Athlete," *Canadian Journal of Applied Physiology* 26 suppl (2001): S186–S191.

12. D.B. Allison et al., "A Novel Soy-based Meal Replacement Formula for Weight Loss Among Obese Individuals: A Randomized Controlled Clinical Trial," *European Journal of Clinical Nutrition* 57 (2003): 514–522.

13. S.B. Kritchevsky and D. Kritchevsky, "Egg Consumption and Coronary Heart Disease: An Epidemiologic Overview," *Journal of the American College of Nutrition* 19:5 suppl (2000): 549S–555S.

14. J.C. Hansen, H.S. Pedersen, and G. Mulvad, "Fatty Acids and Antioxidants in the Inuit Diet: Their Role in Ischemic Heart Disease (IHD) and Possible Interactions with Other Dietary Factors: A Review," *Arctic Medical Research* 53 (1994): 4–17.

15. E. Ernst, T. Saradeth, and G. Achhammer, "Omega-3 Fatty Acids and Acute-phase Proteins," *European Journal of Clinical Investigation* 21 (1991): 77–82.

16. K. Nilausen and H. Meinertz, "Lipoprotein(a) and Dietary Proteins: Casein Lowers Lipoprotein(a) Concentrations as Compared with Soy Protein," *American Journal of Clinical Nutrition* 69:3 (1999): 419–425.

17. R.Z. Stolzenberg-Solomon, E.R. Miller 3rd, M.G. Maguire et al., "Association of Dietary Protein Intake and Coffee Consumption with Serum Homocysteine Concentrations in an Older Population," *American Journal of Clinical Nutrition* 69:3 (1999): 467–475.

18. J.D. MacDougall et al., "The Time Course of Elevated Muscle Protein Synthesis Following Heavy Resistance Exercise," *Canadian Journal of Applied Physiology* 20 (1995): 480–486.

19. Steven R. Hertzler and Yeonsee Kim, "Glycemic and Insulinemic Responses to Energy Bars of Differing Macronutrient Composition in Healthy Adults," *Medical Science Monitor* 9:2 (2003): CR84–90.

20. S. Liu et al., "A Prospective Study of Dietary Glycemic Load, Carbohydrate Intake, and Risk of Coronary Heart Disease in U.S. Women," *American Journal of Clinical Nutrition* 71 (2000): 1455–1461.

21. P.L. Zock, R. Urgert, P.J. Hulshof, and M.B. Katan, "Dietary Trans-fatty Acids: A Risk Factor for Coronary Disease," *Nederlands Tijdschrift voor Geneeskunde* 142:30 (1998): 1701–1704.

Chapter 6: Special Nutritional Needs During Exercise

1. S.N. Steen, *Nutrition for Young Athletes* (Eureka, CA: Nutrition Dimension Inc., 2001).

2. Ibid.

3. Ibid.

4. Ibid.

5. Ibid.

6. Ibid.

Chapter 7: Tips for Gaining and Losing Weight

1. B.A. Dennison et al., “Television Viewing and Television in Bedroom Associated with Overweight Risk among Low-income Preschool Children,” *Pediatrics* 109 (2002): 1028–1035.

2. National Eating Disorders Association, 603 Stewart Street, Suite 803, Seattle, WA 98101; 206-382-3587; www.nationaleatingdisorders.org.

3. Ibid.

Index

I

J

K

L

M

About the Authors

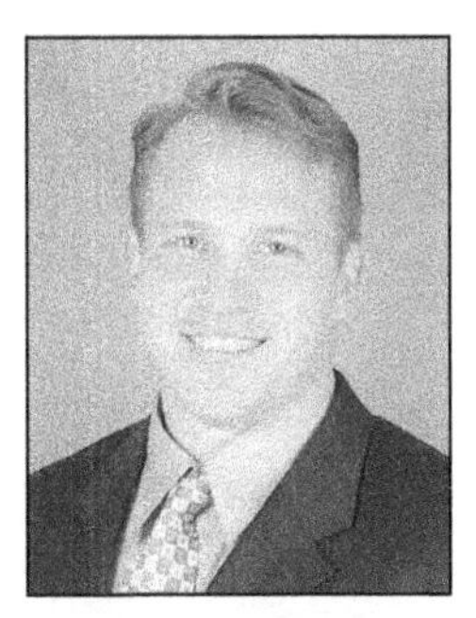

Jeffrey R. Stout earned his Ph.D. in exercise physiology from the University of Nebraska-Lincoln. He has scientific publications in the areas of sports nutrition, muscle fatigue, and the impact of sports participation on growth and development in youth. Dr. Stout was recently awarded the Outstanding Young Investigator Award and the Editorial Excellence Award by the National Strength and Conditioning Association. Furthermore, he is a certified strength and conditioning specialist and Fellow of the American College of Sports Medicine.

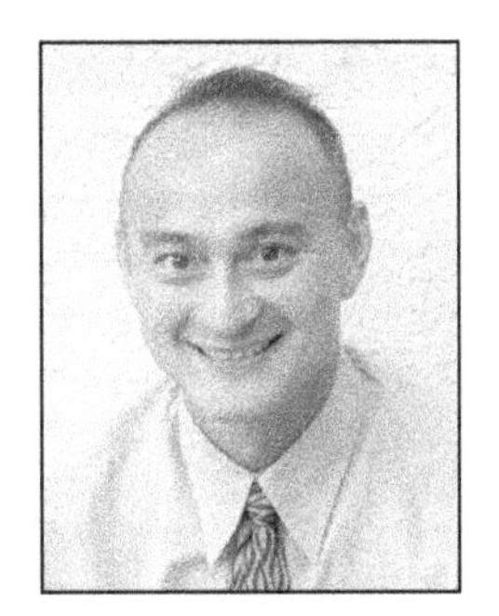

Jose Antonio earned his Ph.D. in the area of muscle physiology and plasticity from the University of Texas Southwestern Medical Center in Dallas Texas and completed a post-doctoral fellowship (at UT Southwestern) in Endocrinology and Metabolism. He is a Fellow of the American College of Sports Medicine and a certified strength and conditioning specialist. Dr. Antonio currently teaches at Florida Atlantic University. He is also one of the founders of the International Society of Sports Nutrition, the only academic society dedicated to promoting the science and practice of sports nutrition.

Dr. Antonio has written for popular magazines such as *Men's Health, Men's Fitness, Muscle & Fitness, Flex, Muscle Media, Energy, Muscle & Fitness Hers, Physical, Running Times,* and *Testosterone.* He has also served as the Adjunct Health and Science Editor of *Muscle & Fitness* and is currently the Editor-in-Chief of *STRONG Research* magazine (www.strong-research.com).

In the scientific arena, he has published more than forty peer-reviewed scientific papers. He has co-authored or co-edited five sports nutrition books with Dr. Jeffrey Stout: *Supplements for Strength-Power Athletes* and *Supplements for Endurance Athletes* (Human Kinetics, 2002), *Sports Supplement Encyclopedia* (Nutricia, 2002), and *Sports Supplements* (Lippincott Williams & Wilkins, 2001).

www.ingramcontent.com/pod-product-compliance
Lightning Source LLC
Jackson TN
JSHW011404130125
77033JS00023B/834

* 9 7 8 1 5 9 1 2 0 0 9 9 4 *